ACTIVE
ISOLATED
STRETCHING

by
Aaron L. Mattes, MS., R.K.T., L.M.T.
Registered Kinesiotherapist and Licensed Massage Therapist
Sarasota, FL

Published By:
Aaron L Mattes
2932 Lexington St.
Sarasota, FL 34231-6118

Photos by Shary Connella and David Johnston

Published By: Aaron L. Mattes
               2932 Lexington Street
               Sarasota, FL 34231

If you are unable to order this book from your local
bookseller, you may order directly from the publisher:
               Call: (941) 922-1939
               Fax: (941) 927-6121

ISBN 0-9656396-0-6

Printed in the United States of America

DEDICATION

To my Mother, Dorothy Mattes, whose shining example has been my guiding light for more than fifty years, to my sons, Lance and Troy, who motivate me to keep progressing; and to my wonderful wife Judy for the past twenty-five years of hard work and continuous encouragement.

ACKNOWLEDGEMENTS

A special thanks to Jim Wharton and Phil Wharton whose tireless efforts have helped bring this work to thousands of people here and abroad.

Thanks to my editor, Eleanor K. Sommer, whose patience, enthusiasm, and cheerfulness made this book possible.

Thanks to my capable secretaries, Le Ann Jotham and Debbie Kopp, for their diligent assistance in typing and coordinating many of the efforts necessary in producing the book.

I would like to offer special thanks to my clinical staff for extending themselves on so many occasions: Joe Boynton, Marvin Carver, Steve Ellis, Michael Enright, John Krakowski, Daryl Lamb, Tami Marugg, Brian Murphy, Jose Oliva, Stacey Sievers, Vicki Sparks, and Stacey Tarricone.

I also appreciate the special encouragement from Terry Simes, Judy Walker, Dan and Tekla Ulrich, Iris Burman, Joe Stinnett, Bo Walker, James Henry, and Michael Loomis.

TABLE OF CONTENTS

PREFACE 1

INTRODUCTION 2

PURPOSE OF STRETCHING 3

REASONS FOR LACK OF FLEXIBILITY 4

AN OVERVIEW OF STRETCHING TECHNIQUES 4

BALLISTIC STRETCH 4

PASSIVE STRETCHING 5

STATIC STRETCHING 6

PROPRIOCEPTIVE NEUROMUSCULAR FACILITATION (PNF) STRETCHING 6

WHEN IS STRETCHING IMPORTANT? 7

    WARM UP 7

    WARM DOWN 7

STRETCH REFLEX 8

AN OUTLINE OF IMPORTANT ACTIVE ISOLATED STRETCHING PRINCIPLES 9

ACTIVE ISOLATED STRETCHING CONSIDERATIONS 10

ACTIVE ISOLATED STRETCHING: REHABILITATION MODALITY 11

HIP-BACK STRETCHING PROTOCOL 12

MAJOR ANTERIOR MUSCLES 14

MAJOR POSTERIOR MUSCLES 15

ACTIVE ISOLATED STRETCHING 16

BEFORE YOU BEGIN, REMEMBER: 16

NECK FLEXIBILITY 17

    ANTERIOR SEMI-CIRCLES 17

    FLEXION 17

    HYPEREXTENSION 18

    OBLIQUE HYPEREXTENSION 18

    LATERAL FLEXION: RIGHT 19

    LATERAL FLEXION: FORWARD OBLIQUE RIGHT 19

    ROTATION: RIGHT 20

    LATERAL FLEXION: LEFT 20

    LATERAL FLEXION: FORWARD OBLIQUE LEFT 21

    ROTATION: LEFT 21

NECK FLEXIBILITY: ACTIVE GRAVITY 21

    ANTERIOR SEMI-CIRCLES 22

    HYPEREXTENSION 22

    LATERAL FLEXION: RIGHT 23

    ROTATION: RIGHT 23

    LATERAL FLEXION: LEFT 24

    ROTATION: LEFT 24

    FLEXION 25

SHOULDER FLEXIBILITY 26

    CIRCUMDUCTION 26

HORIZONTAL ABDUCTION...27

HYPEREXTENSION (OPEN AND WITH HANDS CLASPED)..27

ROTATOR CUFF STRETCHES...28

EXTERNAL ROTATION..28

INTERNAL ROTATION...29

HORIZONTAL FLEXION I..29

HORIZONTAL FLEXION II...30

DELTOID STRETCH...30

TRICEPS STRETCH...30

FORWARD ELEVATION..31

SIDEWARD ELEVATION...31

POSTERIOR HAND CLASP (APLEY SCRATCH TEST)...32

ELBOW, RADIAL-UNLAR, WRIST, FINGER, AND THUMB FLEXIBILITY.................................33

ELBOW FLEXOR STRETCH..33

TRICEPS STRETCH...33

RADIAL-ULNAR PRONATION...34

RADIAL-ULNAR SUPINATION..34

WRIST EXTENSION: PRONE...35

WRIST EXTENSION: SUPINE..35

WRIST FLEXION...36

FINGER EXTENSOR STRETCH..36

FINGER FLEXOR STRETCH..37

FINGER-WRIST FLEXOR STRETCH...37

FINGER ADDUCTOR (WEB) STRETCH..38

THUMB STRETCHING...38

THUMB OPPOSITION STRETCH...38

THUMB ADDUCTOR (WEB) STRETCH..39

THUMB ABDUCTOR STRETCH...39

THUMB EXTENSOR STRETCH..39

HIP FLEXIBILITY...40

BENT KNEE HAMSTRING STRETCH..40

BENT KNEE "INNER HAMSTRING STRETCH"...40

BENT KNEE "OUTER HAMSTRING STRETCH"..41

HAMSTRING STRETCH: BENT KNEE SEATED...41

STRAIGHT LEG HAMSTRING STRETCH...42

STRAIGHT LEG "INNER HAMSTRING STRETCH"...42

STRAIGHT LEG "OUTER HAMSTRING STRETCH"...43

HAMSTRING STRETCH: STRAIGHT LEGS, SEATED...43

HAMSTRING STRETCH: STANDING..44

PSOAS STRETCH: PRONE...44

PSOAS STRETCH: SIDE LYING...45

PSOAS STRETCH: KNEELING..45

PSOAS STRETCH: SUPINE...46

RECTUS FEMORIS STRETCH: SIDE LYING...46

RECTUS FEMORIS STRETCH: STANDING..47

HIP EXTERNAL ROTATOR STRETCH: PRONE...47

HIP EXTERNAL ROTATOR STRETCH: SUPINE...48

HIP EXTERNAL ROTATOR STRETCH WITH ROPE: SEATED..48

HIP EXTERNAL ROTATOR STRETCH WITH HAND: SEATED..49

HIP INTERNAL ROTATOR STRETCH: PRONE..49

HIP INTERNAL ROTATOR STRETCH WITH ROPE: SEATED...50

HIP INTERNAL ROTATOR STRETCH WITH HAND: SEATED..50

HIP INTERNAL ROTATOR STRETCH: SUPINE...51
HIP ABDUCTOR STRETCH...51
HIP ADDUCTOR STRETCH (GROIN)..52
HIP ADDUCTOR STRETCH (GROIN): SEATED...53
HIP FLEXION...53
LATERAL GLUTEUS MAXIMUS STRETCH...54
PIRIFORMIS; FIGURE 4 ROTATOR STRETCH..54

TRUNK FLEXIBILITY 55
SINGLE LEG PELVIC TILT..55
DOUBLE LEG PELVIC TILT...55
REVERSE CURL..56
TRUNK EXTENSION...56
THORACIC EXTENSION...57
UPPER TRUNK EXTENSION..57
UPPER TRUNK EXTENSION: OBLIQUE..58
BENT KNEE TRUNK FLEXION...58
ADVANCED TRUNK ROTATION..59
THORACIC-LUMBAR ROTATION..59
LATERAL TRUNK FLEXION (SEATED OR STANDING)...60
OBLIQUE LATERAL TRUNK FLEXION...60

ANKLE-FOOT FLEXIBILITY 61
DORSAL ANKLE STRETCH 61
SOLEUS STRETCH...62
ACHILLES TENDON STRETCH...62
GASTROCNEMIUS (CALF) STRETCH..63
OUTER GASTROCNEMIUS STRETCH..63
INNER GASTROCNEMIUS STRETCH..63
EVERTOR STRETCH..64
INVERTOR STRETCH..64
FOOT PRONATOR STRETCH..65
FOOT SUPINATOR STRETCH..65
METATARSAL ARCH STRETCH..66
GREAT (BIG) TOE STRETCH (FLEXORS)...67
GREAT (BIG) TOE STRETCH (EXTENSORS)...67
GREAT (BIG) TOE STRETCH (ADDUCTORS)..68
LITTLE TOE STRETCH...69

ASSISTED ACTIVE ISOLATED STRETCHING 71

NECK FLEXIBILITY: ASSISTED...71

NECK STRETCHING: ASSISTED GRAVITY 71
CERVICAL HYPEREXTENSION...72
CERVICAL LATERAL FLEXION: RIGHT...72
CERVICAL ROTATION: RIGHT...73
CERVICAL LATERAL FLEXION: LEFT..73
CERVICAL ROTATION: LEFT..74
CERVICAL FLEXION: SUPINE..74

NECK STRETCHING: ASSISTED: STANDING 75
ANTERIOR SEMI-CIRCLES..75
CERVICAL FLEXION...75
CERVICAL EXTENSION..76
CERVICAL LATERAL FLEXION...76

CERVICAL ROTATION...77

CERVICAL ANTERIOR OBLIQUE..77

CERVICAL POSTERIOR OBLIQUE..78

SHOULDER FLEXIBILITY: ASSISTED...79

SHOULDER CIRCUMDUCTION...79

HORIZONTAL EXTENSION I...79

HORIZONTAL EXTENSION II..80

SHOULDER HYPEREXTENSION: SINGLE ARMS..80

SHOULDER HYPEREXTENSION: HANDS CLASPED.................................80

HORIZONTAL EXTENSION: POSTERIOR..81

SHOULDER: EXTERNAL ROTATION..81

SHOULDER EXTERNAL ROTATION: PRONE...82

SHOULDER EXTERNAL ROTATION: SUPINE..82

SHOULDER: INTERNAL ROTATION...83

SHOULDER INTERNAL ROTATION: PRONE..83

SHOULDER INTERNAL ROTATION: SUPINE...84

HORIZONTAL FLEXION I..84

HORIZONTAL FLEXION II...85

TRICEPS STRETCH: ASSISTED...85

SHOULDER: FORWARD ELEVATION...86

SHOULDER: FORWARD ELEVATION: PRONE...86

SHOULDER: SIDEWARD ELEVATION..87

POSTERIOR HAND CLASP...87

HIP JOINT FLEXIBILITY: ASSISTED..88

HAMSTRING STRETCH: BENT KNEE...88

BICEPS FEMORIS STRETCH: DISTAL...88

SEMITENDINOSUS-SEMIMEMBRANOSUS STRETCH DISTAL..................89

HAMSTRING STRETCH: STRAIGHT LEG...89

SEMITENDINOSUS-SEMIMEMBRANOSUS STRETCH: PROXIMAL..........90

BICEPS FEMORIS STRETCH: PROXIMAL...90

LATERAL HIP-THIGH STRETCH...90

HIP ADDUCTOR (GROIN) STRETCH: SINGLE...91

PSOAS STRETCH..92

QUADRICEPS RECTUS FEMORIS STRETCH: SIDE-LYING........................92

RECTUS FEMORIS: PRONE...93

HIP EXTERNAL ROTATOR STRETCH: PRONE...94

HIP EXTERNAL ROTATOR STRETCH: SUPINE..94

HIP EXTERNAL ROTATOR STRETCH: SITTING...95

HIP INTERNAL ROTATOR STRETCH: PRONE...96

HIP INTERNAL ROTATOR STRETCH: SUPINE..96

HIP INTERNAL ROTATOR STRETCH: SEATED..97

GLUTEUS MAXIMUS STRETCH...97

FIGURE 4 ROTATOR (PIRIFORMIS) STRETCH...98

MEDIAL HIP-THIGH MUSCLE STRETCH...98

TRUNK FLEXIBILITY: ASSISTED...99

SINGLE LEG PELVIC TILT...99

DOUBLE LEG PELVIC TILT...99

BENT KNEE TRUNK FLEXION..100

LUMBAR-SACRAL SPINE STRETCH...100

LUMBAR-SACRAL SPINE STRETCH...101

ADVANCED TRUNK ROTATION..101

THORACIC-LUMBAR ROTATION...102

LATERAL TRUNK FLEXION (STANDING OR SEATED) 103

THORACIC EXTENSION 104

ANKLE-FOOT FLEXIBILITY: ASSISTED 105

SOLEUS STRETCH: PRONE 105

SOLEUS STRETCH: SUPINE 105

ACHILLES STRETCH: PRONE 106

ACHILLES STRETCH: SUPINE 106

GASTROCNEMIUS (CALF) STRETCH 107

ANKLE INVERTOR STRETCH 107

ANKLE EVERTOR STRETCH..108

FOOT PRONATOR STRETCH 108

FOOT SUPINATOR STRETCH] 109

DORSAL ANKLE STRETCH 109

METATARSAL ARCH STRETCH: EXTENSORS 110

METATARSAL ARCH STRETCH: FLEXORS...110

GREAT (BIG) TOE STRETCH (FLEXORS) 111

GREAT (BIG) TOE STRETCH (EXTENSORS) 111

GREAT (BIG) TOE STRETCH (ADDUCTORS) 112

LITTLE TOE STRETCH 113

CONTRAINDICATED OR QUESTIONABLE STRETCHING TECHNIQUES 115

HURDLE STRETCH: FORWARD FLEXION 115

HURDLE STRETCH - HIP FLEXOR 115

FRONT SPLITS...116

GROIN SINGLE LEG 116

LATERAL SPLIT 116

HAMSTRINGS 116

TOE TOUCHING 117

BILLIG STRETCH..117

CALF STRETCH 117

BANANA OR ROCKER STRETCH 117

REVERSE TRUNK FLEXION 118

BACK STRETCH: SEATED 118

NECK BRIDGE 118

HIP ADDUCTOR STRETCH...118

GLOSSARY 119

BIBLIOGRAPHY 122

PREFACE

Human movement is more enjoyable when the body is flexible and capable of performing without restriction. No where is this potential flexibility more apparent than when we watch little children place their toes to their mouths or their legs behind their heads. Such agility reminds us that our flexibility is far less than it once was. One way to regain this flexibility is to regularly practice flexibility exercises. Stretching has been popularized through sports and through activities such as dance, exercise classes, television fitness programs, video cassettes, yoga classes, and books and publications. Therapeutic exercise also plays a crucial role in the treatment of disease or injury, and specific exercises have significant impact in preventive medicine.

Through my work with thousands of people — including Olympic champions; professional, college, and high school athletes; youth sports leagues; and adult amateur athletes — I also have found that the vast majority know painfully little about the proper methods of stretching. I have found that flexibility varies considerably between individuals of the same age.
Although I urge everyone to stretch either to enhance athletic performance or simply to stay healthy, stretching incorrectly can cause more harm than benefit. Stretching should be a painless, peaceful experience. Active people understand the importance of good health and seek methods to improve their abilities by including stretching techniques into their daily schedules. But, even those who are ill or who have been inactive for a period of time can discover the body's capacity for recovery by engaging in flexibility and strength building exercises. Because stretching is adjustable to each individual, there is a stretching program for you whether you are active or inactive.

Movement also helps relieve symptoms of stress. In today's rapidly moving society, stress touches all of our lives. Gentle relaxed stretching movements can invigorate the circulatory, respiratory, and neuromuscular systems, which can alleviate many of the symptoms of stress.

With so many reasons for the addition of stretching to one's daily routine, I have created this book as a guide to teaching the specific methods of isolated stretching exercises, both active and active-assisted. Active Isolated Stretching (AIS) is a result of my twenty-five years of laboratory research; experimentation; and experience in clinical treatment, sports medicine, and teaching. During this time, I have refined and added to these techniques on a regular basis, and I have continued updating this work.
One of the models that has helped me persevere in developing better techniques are the words of the great inventor and industrialist, Henry Ford: "Thinking always ahead, thinking of always trying to do more, brings a state of mind in which nothing seems impossible." This statement has become part of my personal philosophy in which I believe that exceptional skill in performing a procedure is an art and knowledge evolved and formulated in the search for truth is a science.

The influence of Robert E. Shelton, Professor Emeritus of Physical Education, University of Illinois, contributed greatly, both directly and indirectly, to the evolution of my basic theory for teaching musculoskeletal evaluation and flexibility techniques.

This book has been produced not only to illustrate how an individual can stretch properly, but it is also designed to show how an individual may be trained to safely assist others in the stretching process. Doctors, therapists, exercise physiologists, athletic trainers, personal trainers, and athletic coaches should find these techniques, especially those in the active-assisted section, effective for training, injury prevention, and rehabilitation.

INTRODUCTION

FLEXIBILITY, the common synonym for joint range of motion, is a major consideration in sports ability, physical fitness, comfortable posture, and physical medicine. Range of motion components include joints, ligaments, muscles, tendons, fascia, and connective tissue. An understanding of anatomic structures and their limitations is helpful in order to avoid straining these body parts through exercise, athletic endeavors, even daily activities.

Good health should be the number one priority of every human being, and flexibility is an important adjunct to build and maintain optimum health. Even animals can be seen stretching before movement. Prevention of postural problems and joint injuries should be a major goal for everyone. Physical and mental health may be improved with a carefully constructed program of mild stretching exercises, which can help promote wellness through increasing tissue elasticity and joint range of motion.

Motivation to initiate a preventive flexibility program begins with the responsibility of a knowledge-able, caring instructor. Soreness, injury, and lack of positive results can dampen enthusiasm to continue a stretching program. Careful, ongoing instruction helps to insure beneficial results, which are, in my opinion, the greatest source of motivation.

Flexibility is related to body type, sex, age, bone and joint structure, medical history, and other factors beyond an individual's control. (A note of interest: Studies show that girls and women, on the aver-age, are more flexible than males at the same age.) The primary obstacles to flexibility are the musculature and fascia surrounding a specific joint. If the muscles, tendons, and connective tissue surrounding a joint are encouraged to elongate on a regular basis, normal joint range of motion will be retained.

A comprehensive review of literature on the physiology of flexibility (Rasch and Burke 1967; Holland 1968) indicates that flexibility is not a general factor but is specific to each joint. Even the two joints of a bilateral pair in the same individual may display considerable variance. Sedentary living habits and the repeated (habitual) use of flexor muscles are often major reasons for lack of complete range of motion. Flexibility exercises for particular areas are necessary when there is insufficient stimulation of the antigravity muscles of the body and or limited involvement of the flexor muscles. These areas include the posterior thigh, anterior hip, lower back, calves, neck, and the pectoral area of the chest.

Work or exercise that causes overuse of the same muscles repeatedly day after day confines joints within a restricted range of motion and also tends to reduce flexibility. Every activity requires its own unique set of flexibility characteristics, so flexibility developed in one kind of exercise may not be adequate for utilization in another activity. Lack of normal flexibility constrains the extent and quality of performance and contributes to certain ailments.

PURPOSE OF STRETCHING

1. To increase and maintain complete range of motion of the joint.

2. To relieve muscle soreness. Light exercise promotes a better supply of blood and oxygen to the muscles than complete rest and should be pursued unless the injury to muscles or joints precludes further activity.

3. To help improve the capacity for activity. Stretched muscles require less energy for completion of movements.

4. To assist in decreasing unnecessary neuromuscular tension, promote general body relaxation, and reduce emotional stress.

5. To relieve muscle-joint stiffness associated with the aging process.

6. To increase musculotendinous extendibility. Muscle can be stretched 1.6 times its resting length before it tears.

7. To elongate the fascia, which provides the binding together support system to stabilize muscles, organs, and most body tissue. Elasticity varies between individuals and is a major reason some individuals experience slower progress in attaining flexibility.

8. To help prevent joint and muscle strains and tears or the re-injury of these areas.

9. As a major part of the pre-activity warm-up to increase tissue temperature through an increased metabolic rate.

10. As part of the warm-down process to increase blood flow to the fatigued area, eliminate toxic waste products from cells, reduce soreness, increase muscle relaxation, and improve flexibility.

11. To help provide greater potentials for physical and athletic skills.

12. To reduce tightness that may contribute to pain, spasm, or cramping.

13. To provide an important adjunct toward recovery during the process of rehabilitation.

REASONS FOR LACK OF FLEXIBILITY

1. Muscle imbalance. Many times the agonist muscles are far weaker than corresponding antagonist muscles on opposite side of joint. This is particularly true of the overdeveloped muscles of weight trainers who often concentrate on certain muscles without regard to *all* the muscles in a joint. Muscle imbalance may also occur in cases of stroke; cerebral palsy; spasm; and orthopedic spinal conditions such as scoliosis, lordosis or kyphosis. The process of aging also increases the chance of muscle imbalance.

2. The temporary or chronic inability to actively move a joint in a given direction because of paralysis, neurological disease, neurological injury, or joint immobilization.

3. Overuse of the muscle without maintaining complete range of motion. Activities that are constantly performed without stretching will result in tight joints and muscles. Muscles such as the gastrocnemius, rectus femoris, psoas, and hamstrings shorten from continuous stress of activities such as running, jumping, stopping, and starting. Even the regular wearing of high heels or continually running only on the balls of the feet can result in a shortened Achilles tendon or gastrocnemius muscle.

4. Effects of aging. Aging affects tissue elasticity as muscle mass atrophy occurs. Inactivity is a major cause of muscle weakness, which results in hypertonicity (a condition in which the muscle becomes too toned — hard and nonpliable) and inelasticity of less used muscles. Disease, injury, and inactivity causes de-conditioning and progressive loss of muscle mass. Improvement potentials are different at every age and the rate of flexibility development may differ from person to person.

5. Periods of rapid growth. Body coordination is affected during times of growth when the body displays rapid change in height or weight. This is illustrated by a temporary loss of coordination as musculotendinous structure flexibility fails to keep up to the increased long bone or soft tissue growth.

AN OVERVIEW OF *STRETCHING TECHNIQUES*

The following information is an overview of other stretching techniques presented in various journals and books, which describe and illustrate specific instructions. It is not the purpose of this book to criticize other authors and the years of hard work and research they have undertaken, only to present these ideas so the reader has a comparison of other stretching methods.

BALLISTIC STRETCH

Ballistic stretching, the use of bouncing, rebounding, bobbing, or rhythmic motion to increase range of motion, is contraindicated in the program of AIS. Other terms synonymous with "ballistic" are *dynamic, kinetic* or *body momentum*.

Ballistic stretching is sometimes employed in sports such as gymnastics, karate, and dance. An example is the hurdler's stretch, which employs bobbing of the trunk toward an extended leg to stretch the hamstrings. It requires extending the upper body backwards and lying down to stretch the trail leg; a bouncing motion of the trail thigh is used to stretch the quadriceps.

Continued On Following Page

BALLISTIC STRETCH (CON'T.)

Ballistic motion or bouncing is especially contraindicated for extremely weak or paralyzed muscles because the rapid movements activate the muscle spindle resulting in premature involvement of the *stretch reflex* (See detailed explanation of stretch reflex on page 8). Rapid movement can also cause pain and increase the possibility of muscle or tendon rupture.

There are many logical physiological principles that preclude ballistic stretching from being safe and beneficial. Here are a few:

1. Ballistic stretching aggravates muscles and connective tissue because it is difficult to judge the stretch tolerance of the tissues or to control the force of the body momentum;

2. Causes small muscle tears that may produce inflexible scar tissue;

3. Often causes over-tense muscles rather than producing relaxation; and

4. May initiate a "stretch reflex" within the very muscles being stretched, causing rapid contraction of the muscles to be stretched and possibly resulting in spasms.

PASSIVE STRETCHING

Passive stretching is often indicated when an individual is paralyzed or the antagonist muscle group is injured or paralyzed. In passive stretching, the individual makes no contribution or active contraction. If joint range of motion is not maintained following problems such as a stroke or spinal cord injury, the musculotendinous unit will shorten and joint motion will be lost in the opposite direction of the affected muscles.

The use of prolonged (passive) stretching employs a partner who extends the mobility-range gradually to the utmost position. This assistant provides continuous external assistance just below the pain threshold for as long one minute.

Passive stretching should be a slow, steady movement, using gentle force to lengthen the soft tissues. Careful movement of the tissues will help prevent pain to the patient. However, passive stretching has the following limitations:

1. There is dependency on an assistant. A mistake during prolonged stretch can injure the patient, wiping out all the benefits of the flexibility program.

2. Passive stretching may be painful.

3. There is no motor learning and no improvement in the capacity for active motion of the tight muscle or its opponent.

4. Passive stretching fails to activate or strengthen the weak, overstretched agonist opposing the tight muscle(s). When these muscles are activated they help establish a pattern for coordinated motion.

5. When passive stretching occurs too rapidly and with too much force, the stretch reflex initiates contraction of the muscle, defeating the purpose of the procedure.

STATIC STRETCHING

Static stretching or slow stretching has been used for centuries by those involved in yoga. Static stretching has been popularized through television fitness programs, sports, dance, and exercise classes. It is the most widely used method of flexibility training. Static stretching has received international exposure through the work of Bob Anderson and his book, *Stretching*. Anderson's stretching is achieved by applying a low force long duration stretch to improve flexibility. The stretch is divided into two phases:

1. The Easy Stretch: In the Easy Stretch position, which lasts 10 to 30 seconds, you stretch to the point where you feel mild tension and relax as you hold the stretch without bouncing. You find the degree of tension that is comfortable. The Easy Stretch reduces muscular tightness and readies the tissue for the developmental stretch.

2. The Developmental Stretch: The purpose of the Developmental Stretch is to fine tune the muscles and increase flexibility. You move slowly into the Developmental Stretch until you feel a mild tension, and then you hold it from 10 to 30 seconds. You exhale as you bend forward and then breathe rhythmically for the duration of the stretch.

In 1982 Dr. Sven A. Solveborn, a Swedish sports-medicine physician published *The Book About Stretching*. His method employs the Tighten-Relax-Stretch technique.

1. Tighten the muscles with static-isometric muscle tension. Keep the position for 10 to 30 seconds.

2. Relax 2 to 3 seconds.

3. Stretch out the muscle gently, as far as possible. Stay in this position for as long as you can tighten the muscle (10 to 30 seconds).

PROPRIOCEPTIVE NEUROMUSCULAR FACILITATION (PNF) STRETCHING

The Proprioceptive Neuromuscular Facilitation approach developed by L. E. Holt in 1971 utilizes the natural physiological fact that a muscle contraction is normally followed by relaxation of the opposite antagonistic muscle(s). The object of the PNF method is to purposefully stimulate the neural mechanisms of contraction and relaxation.

Active PNF employs motion that is extended as far as possible through active muscle work for six seconds. This is followed by a maximum isometric muscle tightening of the counter-acting muscles and is done with resistance from a practice partner or therapist. This phase is followed by active efforts to stretch the muscle farther. This is interchanged with tightening of the counteracting muscle with resistance in six seconds intervals for one minute.

The complexity of PNF procedures, requires the therapist or assistant to be actively involved with the subject at all times. One must verbally cue the initiation of effort and control the timing of movements, mechanically guiding the movements through the diagonal-spiral path and applying graded resistance matched to the subject's increase in strength of contraction. The experience of the therapist in addition to *strength* of the therapist and the patient determines the success or failure of PNF stretching. This time consuming technique demands the therapeutic capability of sustaining exertion while offering graded resistance to movements.

WHEN IS STRETCHING IMPORTANT?

WARM UP

Warm-up stretching is important to help prevent muscle strain or tears that can occur from sudden over-lengthening of the musculotendinous unit. The primary purpose of a warm-up before physical activity is to raise the deep temperature within the body and to lengthen contracted muscle and fascia fibers. The warm-up time for the specific body parts, can last from 30 to 45 minutes or more, depending on the movements to be performed and the stress and strain of the subsequent activity. The preliminary warm-up should include gentle general exercises; walking, including walking in place, rope jumping, or gentle running in place; or use of the stationary bicycle. This warms the muscles and prepares them for stretching. The most important phase of the warm-up should be specific isolated stretching exercises. During this time tissues are infused with blood, oxygen, and nutrients. The length of time spent on this phase should be commensurate with the stiffness or inflexibility of the joint being stretched. Muscles that serve more than one joint such as the hamstrings, rectus femoris (quadriceps) and the gastrocnemius are primary examples. Muscles such as the shoulder rotator cuff that start or stop joint movements are also vulnerable to injury and require extra stretching.

The age of the individual should also be considered. An older person may require a longer warm-up period than a younger one. It is also important that a person spend time incorporating the primary movements contained in the skills of the sport or activity in prepartion for actually performing the activity. Various studies have shown warm-ups help increase the speed of nerve impulses, which provides greater body movement potentials.

Active Isolated Stretching as warm-ups for the athlete are designed to enhance the athlete's performance, prevent injury, and reduce recovery time. Stretching permits the athlete to train at a higher level without discomfort. Most importantly AIS enhances performance during competition. As record breaking professional football wide receiver Art Monk has stated, "Active Isolated Stretching is the primary reason for a lengthened athletic career."

WARM DOWN

Following vigorous activity, you should allow the body systems to slow down gradually and let the heart rate decrease to pre-exercise levels. Post workout stretching reduces muscular tension and help prevent or delay the onset of muscle soreness and fatigue, which are often caused by body waste fluids that accumulate in the muscle tissues causing stiffness, discomfort, and soreness. Active Isolated Stretching helps maintain tissue homeostasis and a better state of vitality.

After major activity, the following steps are important for maximal recovery in the shortest possible time.

1. Gradually decrease the intensity using slower body motions.
2. This is followed by slow isotonic movements.
3. Incorporate isolated specific stretching movements to decrease waste materials in the tissues, and increase blood flow, oxygen, and nutritional levels to the prefatigue levels as soon as possible. Postactivity stretching also helps decrease the cramping and stiffness associated with fatigue. Be sure to drink plenty of fluids and to practice gentle deep breathing to help return the body to the pre-exercise levels as soon as possible following the activity. Warm downs are also an excellent opportunity to work on flexibility improvement as tissue temperature will be at its highest level. Stretching following performance or a day of work helps promote greater relaxation of the entire body.

STRETCH REFLEX

The *stretch reflex* is a regulatory mechanism of the nervous system that helps enable the body to maintain muscle tone and posture. It is activated as a defensive protection in an attempt to avoid over-stretching and help prevent muscle-tendon injuries. If you do not have adequate flexibility for a required movement, the stretch reflex contraction exerts force against the desired movement, and more energy is required to overcome the stretch reflex force and this increases the possibility of injury. The exercises in this book are based on a continued program of flexibility that avoid the activation of this defensive mechanism. All the stretches in this program are held for a duration of 1 1/2 to 2 seconds. Longer periods of stretch will cause prolonged activation of the stretch reflex.

The major component of the stretch reflex is located in the muscle spindle. The purpose of the muscle spindle is to monitor the velocity and duration of a stretching force that is being applied to a muscle. The spindle is innervated by a gamma motor neuron and is always maintained by some degree of tension even if the muscle is in a shortened position. This ensures the spindle will constantly be ready to monitor the stretch. When it is stretched, the muscle receives a signal to contract, which helps prevent overextension. When the stretch is slow and mild, the force of the contraction triggered by the stretch reflex also will be gentle. If the force of the stretch is hard or bouncing then the contraction will be proportionate to that force, increasing the potential of injury.[1]

Muscle spindles have two kinds of sensory receptors: primary receptors called **annulospiral** wrap around the large (secondary) **intrafusal** fibers at the center regions. Afferent nerve fibers lead from intrafusal fibers and have a fast conduction rate. The afferent impulse connects through neurons in the spinal cord with the muscle's antagonist. The input is responsible for reciprocal innervation of the antagonist, preventing drag of the antagonist on the agonist. The primary receptors have a lower threshold than do the secondary endings and are more sensitive to stretch. This sensitive primary receptor produces a discharge signal known as the *stretch reflex*.

Muscle spindles also have secondary, or flower-spray endings, located at the polar ends of many but not all intrafusal fibers. These secondary endings are believed to be responsible for a flexor reflex with inhibition of the extensor muscles. As a muscle shortens, tension on the muscle spindle decreases.[2] The second component of the stretch reflex are the Golgi tendon organs located at the junction of muscle fibers and their tendinous attachments at both ends of the muscle. They are sensitive to muscle contraction and muscle stretch but cannot distinguish between the two. They discharge as a result of tension in the tendon. This discharge inhibits the muscle and the facilitation of its antagonist. This safety valve action prevents excessive contraction to the muscle so that the opposing muscle group, which is being stretched, will not be hurt by the force of the contraction.[3]
Stretching exercises increase the ability of the tissues to lengthen, enabling joints to move through a greater range before meeting this resistance from tension and muscle contraction activated by the stretch reflex.

[1]Beaulieu, John E., Stretching for all Sports, California: Athletic Press, 1984, p. 38.
[2]Rasch, Philip J., Kinesiology and Applied Anatomy, Lea & Febiger, 1989, p. 70.
[3]Rasch, op. cit., p. 68.

AN OUTLINE OF IMPORTANT ACTIVE ISOLATED STRETCHING PRINCIPLES

1. The three I's for efficient stretching with maximum results:
    a. <u>Identify</u> the specific muscles to be stretched.
    b. <u>Isolate</u> the muscles to be stretched by using precise localized movements. Each individual must employ exactness of detail in order to achieve maximum results.
    c. <u>Intensify</u> the contractile effort of the agonist muscles opposite to the antagonist muscles that are reciprocally relaxing and lengthening on the opposite side of the joint. Reciprocal innervation of the muscles to contract will also simultaneously reciprocally inhibit the opposite side muscle to relax and lengthen.

2. Increase local blood flow, oxygen, and nutrition to tissues before and after activity. The contracting muscles are major vehicles used to deliver blood and oxygen. Repetitive isotonic muscle contractions deliver greater amounts of blood, oxygen and nutrition to specific regions more rapidly than static or isometric muscle contractions. Numerous repetitions are an important consideration in a thorough warm-up or postactivity recovery process.

3. The fuel for muscular action comes from the burning of fatty acids and glucose in the presence of oxygen. The glucose comes from stored muscle fuel (glycogen) and from the blood. If oxygen is lacking, the muscles get energy by converting glucose to lactic acid, a waste product that causes muscles to fatigue. Regular breathing during muscular exertion decreases this fatigue. Breathe regularly and avoid holding your breath — even for short periods. Establish the following breathing rhythm when stretching:
    Exhale during the work phase of stretching;
    Inhale as the body part returns to the starting posture.

4. For maximum safety, stretch the muscles and connective tissue to the degree where the myotatic (stretch) reflex is activated and move beyond to the point of *light* irritation. Stretch gently for 1 1/2 to 2 seconds, release the pressure, return to the starting position, and repeat the prescribed number of repetitions. Releasing the pressure on the tissues being stretched at the point of light irritation helps prevent the reversal contraction of the tissue triggered by the stretch reflex. Intentional violation of the stretch reflex may result in soreness from overstretching or scar tissue from tissue tearing.

5. Stretching is a daily requirement. Muscles shorten, stiffen, or become tense from work, training, posture, gravity, or stress. Tissue can be revitalized by proper nutrition, rest, and exercise. Exercises such as Active Isolated Stretching help restore full joint movement, decrease tissue soreness and fatigue, increase tissue pliability and posture.

6. Overstretched Principle: Range of movement will not be maintained unless the existing limit is reached regularly, nor will it be improved unless that limit is exceeded. Increased flexibility is achieved by properly implementing a movement that exceeds the momentarily existing range of motion.

7. Reversibility: The cessation of regular specific training causes more loss in mobility than other elements such as strength and endurance. Gross flexibility is lost gradually, however specific isolated flexibility should be included as part of the training routine, exercise session, or as a separate specific unit.

Continued On Following Page

8. Comparing And Competing: There is great potential for overstretching in exercise classes and during team flexibility workouts, where a wide range of abilities exists. Individuals should not be competitive when it comes to stretching; instead they should stay tuned to their own bodies. Comparing and competing against others in stretching can lead to soreness and injury.

9. Gradualism: The development of flexibility takes time. Some people develop flexibility rapidly, while others may require many sessions to reach the same level. Set realistic goals for yourself and progress with consistent daily effort.

10. Relaxation: Other than stretching itself, relaxation is the most important factor in developing flexibility. Fatigue results from tension in contracted muscles, inflexibility, insufficient blood and oxygen, and limited nutritional supply to the tissues. The ability to relax is important because it decreases tension, which increases the ability to function effectively and efficiently.

11. Mindset: A positive mental attitude is important. Without a positive mindset, the best possible results cannot be achieved.

ACTIVE ISOLATED STRETCHING CONSIDERATIONS

The expression, "No Pain, No Gain" is a dangerous philosophy in a sound flexibility program. There should never be an injury in a flexibility program. Numerous research articles encourage slow, rhythmical stretching movements which are safest, cause less irritation to the tissues being stretched, require less energy expenditure, and will yield more qualitative relief from muscular distress. A flexibility program to obtain or maintain optimum range of each fundamental joint movement is a long-term undertaking; don't risk injury by rushing the process.

Bouncing, jerking, or prolonged force causes tight tissues to contract increasing the possibility of muscle soreness or microscopic muscle tears initiating the formation of scar tissue, which decreases tissue elasticity. (Sherrington's Law states that a muscle has the potential to contract or relax but cannot do both simultaneously). Any type of movement, such as static stretching, that encourages shortening or lengthening of muscle fibers at both ends simultaneously may cause spasm, pain, or injury. For example, an exercise referred to as the *rocker* or *banana* is performed by lifting the legs, head, and shoulders at the same time, which shortens the back muscles at both ends. Toe touching and the hurdle stretch are also examples of stretches that encourage lengthening contractions of muscle fibers at both origin and insertion by making use of gravity, body weight, or momentum at the terminal point of joint movement. Active Isolated Stretching calls for stretches that isolate the specific parts of the muscles, such as the hamstrings, rectus femoris, or gastrocnemius, that serve more than one joint .

Continued On Following Page

Many of the traditional yoga or static stretching techniques employ isometric eccentric (lengthening) muscle contractions when stretching. Employing such techniques in which working muscles and connective tissues are actively contracting, makes relaxation of muscle tension improbable and may lead to major soreness or injury. Stretching should always allow for the greatest possible safety considerations. The stretch reflex should be used as a primary safety precaution. The AIS method employs the contracting muscles opposite to the muscles that are to be lengthened as the movement force (agonist contracts, antagonist relaxes).

In AIS where the use of external force is appropriate, use your hands or a rope to provide assistance and gentle stretch. The use of partners in a stretching program must be administered very carefully. Inexperienced assistants may move the joint too far which can result in soreness or injury. Careful consideration and close communication provides maximum effectiveness without endangering the participant. The section in this book on Assisted Active Isolated Stretching illustrates the exercises and principles to be considered.

Stretching should be a daily practice. Flexibility is one of the most important aspects of conditioning for an athlete, and stretching exercises should be performed prior to any athletic performance or strength training session. It is advisable to do a minimum of 20 to 30 minutes of isolated stretching prior to vigorous participation. For those not involved in athletics, a minimum of 15 to 20 minutes of gentle stretching should be practiced on a daily basis to maintain good posture and tissue elasticity. Early morning stretching warms the body in preparation for physical stresses such as those produced by gravity, postures, or lifting. Stretching can also be used as a means of relaxation or restoration at the end of a work day or following activity.

In the following chapters which detail the AIS program, stretching exercises are presented which isolate each muscle or group of muscles that provide a specific joint movement. These exercises have been used successfully by thousands of people for tension reduction; injury prevention; improvement of sports performance; and restoration of range of movement in rehabilitation following surgery, injury, or other conditions that could result in the loss of flexibility. Be exacting in the application of the stretching exercises. Compensation through the improper form, infrequent application of the exercises, lack of effort, and incorrect technique will result in problems such as soreness, injury, or lack of improvement.

ACTIVE ISOLATED STRETCHING: REHABILITATION MODALITY

Active Isolated Stretching can be used in rehabilitation and restoration to assist in recovery of an acute problem or to keep a chronic problem from becoming acute. Appropriate and accurate stretching helps a person recover faster and with less discomfort, i.e., muscles spasms or articulatory stiffness. When AIS is used following irritation from overworked and stressed muscles, patients experience rapid recovery with less tension and depression.

Consistent use of AIS helps prevent trigger points and biomechanical stress, which can relieve tender areas before they become a problem. Active Isolated Stretching also helps create a soft, pliable scar tissue and aids in the reduction of swelling, edema, and bruising. Using repeated muscle contractions further activates the lymphatic system, aids in lung ventilation, promotes the removal of toxins and acids, builds additional capillaries, nourishes and lubricates the muscles.

HIP-BACK STRETCHING PROTOCOL

Because lower back problems are among the most common complaints or patients, I have developed the following protocol specifically to promote hip flexibility and strength, which in my opinion is vital to a strong, healthy, and flexible back.

Problems with the hip can result in scoliosis or a "long leg-short leg" status with accompanying pelvic hike, tilt ,or rotation. Many other back and hip ailments have their origin in muscle imbalance. The following list of AIS exercises have been instrumental in alleviating many of those problems. For maximum results perform these exercises in the order presented. Initially, Assisted AIS is helpful in releasing these inflexible tissues.

	Active Page	Assisted Page
1. Single Leg Pelvic Tilt	55	99
2. Double Leg Pelvic Tilt	55	99
3. Hamstring Stretch - Bent Knee	40	88
4. Hamstring Stretch - Straight Leg	42	89
5. Hip Adductor Stretch	52	91
6. Hip Abductor Stretch	51	90
7. Psoas Stretch	45	92
8. Rectus Femoris Stretch	46	92
9. Lateral Hip Rotators	48	94
10. Medial Hip Rotators	51	96
11. Gluteus Maximus Stretch	54	97
12. Biceps Femoris Stretch	43	90
13. Piriformis Stretch	54	98
14. Medial Hip Rotators - Supine	51	98
15. Bent Knee Trunk Flexion	58	100
16. Advanced Trunk Rotation	59	101
17. Thoracic - Lumbar Rotation	59	102
18. Lateral Trunk Flexion	60	103
19. Lateral Trunk Flexion Oblique	60	103
20. Gastrocnemius (calf) Stretch	63	107

MAJOR ANTERIOR MUSCLES

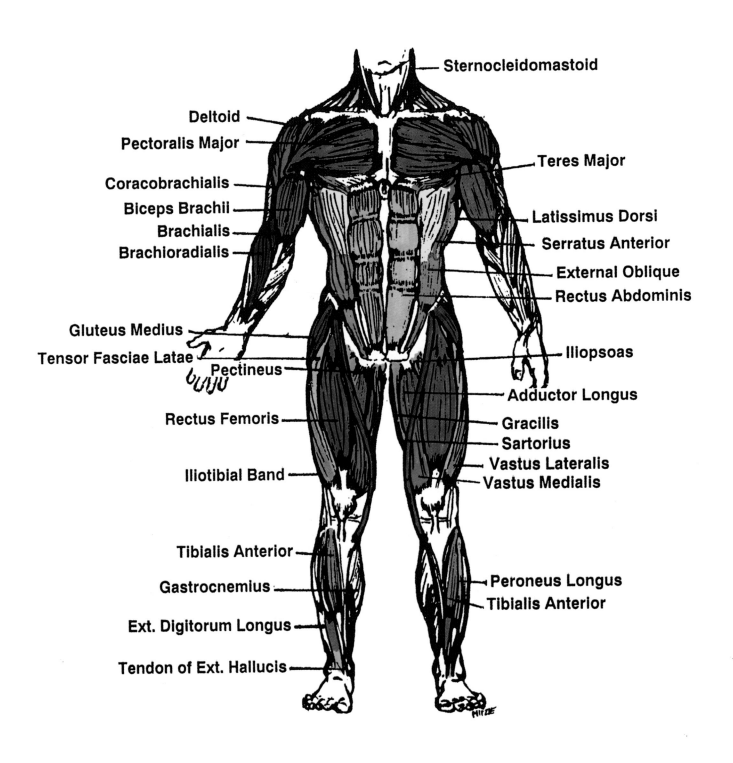

Sternocleidomastoid

Deltoid

Pectoralis Major

Teres Major

Coracobrachialis

Biceps Brachii

Latissimus Dorsi

Brachialis

Serratus Anterior

Brachioradialis

External Oblique

Rectus Abdominis

Gluteus Medius

Tensor Fasciae Latae

Iliopsoas

Pectineus

Adductor Longus

Rectus Femoris

Gracilis

Sartorius

Vastus Lateralis

Iliotibial Band

Vastus Medialis

Tibialis Anterior

Peroneus Longus

Gastrocnemius

Tibialis Anterior

Ext. Digitorum Longus

Tendon of Ext. Hallucis

MAJOR POSTERIOR MUSCLES

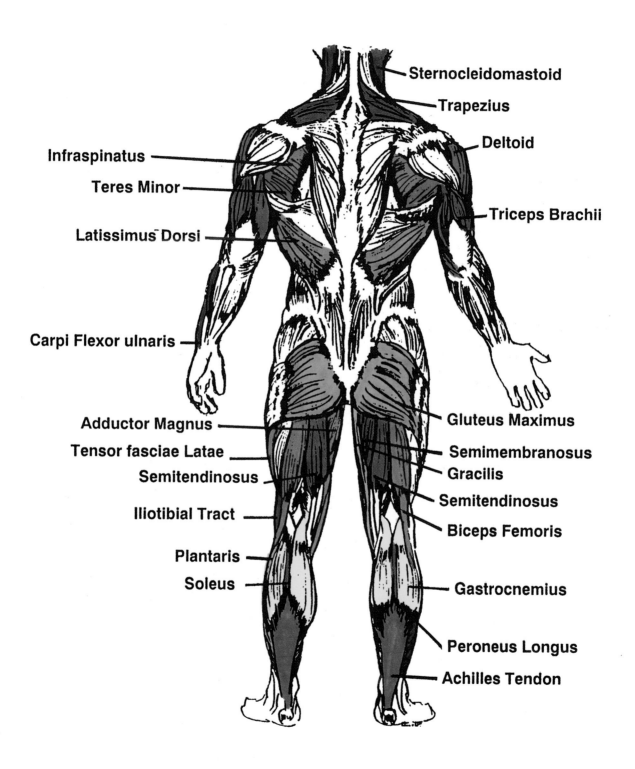

Sternocleidomastoid

Trapezius

Deltoid

Infraspinatus

Teres Minor

Triceps Brachii

Latissimus Dorsi

Carpi Flexor ulnaris

Gluteus Maximus

Adductor Magnus

Semimembranosus

Tensor fasciae Latae

Gracilis

Semitendinosus

Semitendinosus

Iliotibial Tract

Biceps Femoris

Plantaris

Soleus

Gastrocnemius

Peroneus Longus

Achilles Tendon

ACTIVE ISOLATED STRETCHING

BEFORE YOU BEGIN, REMEMBER:

- Active Isolated Stretching is an important part of warm up, warm down, training, or rehabilitation.
- Specificity is important to achieve maximum circulation, relaxation, and tissue elongation. *Identify* the muscles to be stretched; then *isolate* those muscles by using precise, localized movements; and finally *intensify* the movement with assistance of your hand or a rope.
- Never stretch the lengthened tissues more than 1 1/2 to 2 seconds and then release to starting (neutral) position.
- Always return the area being stretched to the starting position before continuing to the prescribed repetitions.
- Always exhale during the stretching phase and inhale during the recovery phase (as you return to the starting position).
- Monitor the stretch reflex carefully as the tissue is stretched to the point of light irritation, then release the tension to prevent reversal contraction of the tissue being stretched.

As you examine the exercises in the following chapters, you will see that there are a variety of detailed and specific exercises for AIS and Assisted AIS techniques that can increase tissue-joint movement and improve physiological function without the pain or injury potenial that exists in many programs.

Noted author, lecturer and TV health authority Dr. Robert Arnot, MD, couldn't have made it clearer in these comments about his recent book, *Dr. Bob Arnot's Guide to Turning back the Clock*. He was tempted, he says, *not* to include a chapter on stretching because, as with many people, he never achieved anything worthwhile with traditional stretching. However, Dr. Arnot says he found that his "muscles and joints were easily unchained with AIS stretching. The body workload is removed allowing freedom of movement."

And so in a book by one of the world's leading health authorities, you will find a chapter that supports and encourages AIS as a vital component not only for success in sports but for a healthy lifestyle as well.

NECK FLEXIBILITY

Standing or sitting

These movement are designed to insure maximum range of motion for injury prevention in sports and to generally improve range of motion and provide relief of cervical muscle tension. The standing or sitting neck flexibility series allows you to move your head in a given direction actively and to assist the movement with your hands.

ANTERIOR SEMI-CIRCLES

Introduction: Full circumduction places unwarranted stress on tendons and ligaments and is contraindicated for those suffering from whiplash, post fracture, or disc problems. Semi-circumduction, however, is a gentle general warm-up exercise that increases circulation prior to the specific fundamental movements of the neck.

Method: Employ a relaxed semi-circular motion moving the head in pendular movements from side to side. Move head in half circles. Begin by lowering head toward sternum (breast bone). Move chin toward top of one shoulder, and then lower chin toward breast bone and move to opposite shoulder. Repeat movement in opposite direction.

Repetitions: 8-10

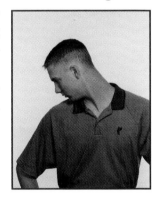 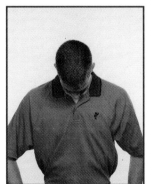 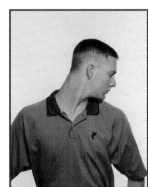

FLEXION

Muscles Stretched: Cervical extensor muscles including the multifidus, semispinalis, oblique capitus, and erector spinae.

Muscles Contracted: Anterior cervical flexor muscles, including the rectus capitus anterior, rectus capitis lateralis, sternocleidomastoid, longus colli, longus capitis, and scalene muscles.

Method: Tuck chin as close to neck as possible, assist terminal (last) movement with hands on back of head. Release and return to neutral position.

Compensation Check: Do not allow spinal areas below the neck to bend downward as head moves forward.

Repetitions: 8-10

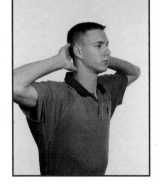 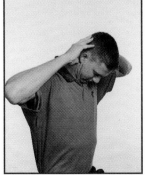

HYPEREXTENSION

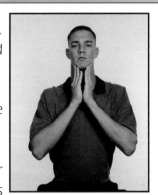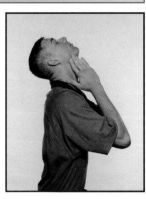

Muscles Stretched: Cervical flexors, including the longus colli, longus capitis, rectus capitis anterior, rectus capitis lateralis, and scalene muscles.

Muscles Contracted: Extensor muscles including the multifidus, semispinalis, oblique capitus, and erector spinae.

Method: Extend head backward by contracting the extensor muscles. Assist at the end of the movement with the hands under the outer borders of the jaw or on the forehead. Do not extend spinal areas below the neck. Stretch the flexor muscles. Release to the neutral position and repeat.

Notes: For those with disc involvement or following whiplash or severe trauma, hyperextension is more appropriately performed in a prone position. (See Neck Flexibility: Active Gravity).

Repetitions: 8-10

OBLIQUE HYPEREXTENSION

Muscles Stretched: Anterior scalenus, sternocleidomastoid, longus colli cervicus, longus capitus, and rectus capitus muscles.

Method: To lengthen these muscles, rotate head 45 degrees then extend neck backwards at 45 degree angle. Move head (ear) towards outer border of scapula in direction head is rotated. Assist movement gently with same side hand. Return to neutral position. Rotate head in opposite direction and move ear toward outer shoulder blade.

Compensation Check: Do not arch back.

Repetitions: 8-10

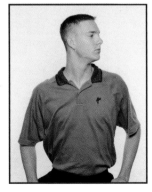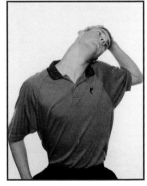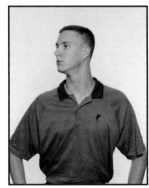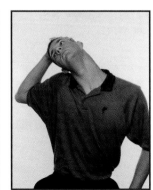

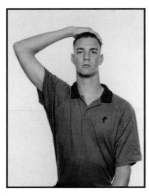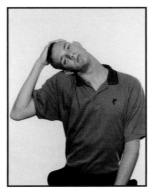

Muscles Stretched: Left lateral muscles, including the scalene muscles sternocleidomastoid, sacrospinous, and splenius capitis muscles.

Muscles Contracted: Right cervical lateral flexors.

Method: To stretch the lateral muscles on the left side of the neck contract the same cervical lateral flexors on the right side of the neck. Move head to the right (ear downward toward shoulder) and, at end of movement, assist with right hand placed on left side of head. Focus on object directly in front of eyes to prevent movement out of correct frontal plane. Stretch and return to neutral position.

Compensation Check: Do not shrug left shoulder or bend mid (thoracic) and lower (lumbar) spine laterally.

Repetitions: 8-10

LATERAL FLEXION: FORWARD OBLIQUE RIGHT

Muscles Stretched: Upper trapezius and levator scapula semispinalis capitis, longissimus capitis, erector spinae, and middle posterior scalene muscles.

Muscles Contracted: Right side sternocleidomastoid and pre-vertebral muscles.

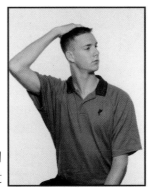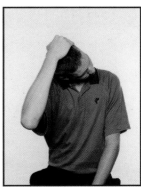

Method: Rotate head 45 degrees to the left, then move head at 45 degree angle towards right breast by contracting right side sternocleidomastoid and prevertebral muscles. Assist movement with right hand.

Compensation Check: Do not elevate left shoulder or lateral flex trunk to the right.

Repetitions: 8-10

ROTATION: RIGHT

Muscles Stretched: Left cervical rotators, including the multifidus, rotators, semispinalis, and sternocleidomastoid muscles.

Muscles Contracted: Right cervical rotators.

Method: Rotate head to the right by contracting the same right side cervical rotators. Assist at end of movement by placing right hand along left side of mandible (jaw) and left hand on right side of head toward back end. Stretch and release to neutral position.

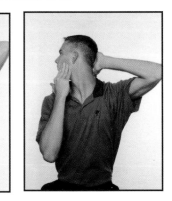

Compensation Check: Do not allow compensation by shrugging shoulders or rotating upper trunk.

Repetitions: 8-10

LATERAL FLEXION: LEFT

Muscles Stretched: Right lateral muscles of the neck including the scalene muscles, sternocleidomastoid, sacrospinous, and splenius capitis muscles.

Muscles Contracted: Left cervical lateral flexors.

Method: Move head to the left (ear downward toward shoulder). Assist at end of movement with left hand placed on right side of head. Focus on an object directly in front of your eyes to prevent movement out of correct frontal plane. Stretch and return to neutral position.

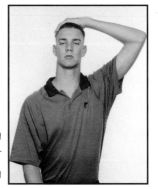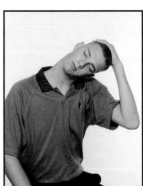

Compensation Check: Do not shrug right shoulder or bend mid spine (thoracic) and lower spine (lumbar) laterally.

Repetitions: 8-10

LATERAL FLEXION: FORWARD OBLIQUE LEFT

Muscles Stretched: Upper trapezius and levator scapula semispinalis capitis, longissimus capitis, erector spinae, and middle posterior scalene muscles.

Muscles Contracted: Left side sternocleidomastoid and prevertebral muscles.

Method: Rotate head 45 degrees to the right. Move head at 45 degree angle towards left breast by contracting left side sternocleidomastoid and prevertebral muscles. Assist movement with left hand. Return to starting position and repeat.

Repetitions: 8-10

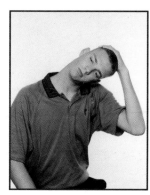

ROTATION: LEFT

Muscles Stretched: Right side neck rotators, including the multifidus, rotators, semispinalis, and sternocleidomastoid muscles.

Muscles Contracted: Left side cervical rotators.

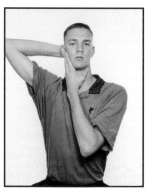 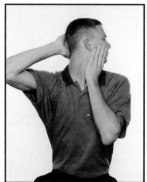

Method: Rotate head to the left by contracting opposite side (left) cervical rotators. Assist at end of movement by placing left hand along right side of mandible (jaw) and right hand on left side of head towards back end.

Compensation Check: Do not allow compensation by shrugging shoulders or rotating upper trunk. Stretch and release to neutral position.

Repetitions: 8-10

NECK FLEXIBILITY: ACTIVE GRAVITY

Introduction:
Proper warming of neck musculature and maintaining normal joint range of motion may help reduce muscle strain and the possibility of severe injury such as nerve damage, fracture, or paralysis. This is especially important in sports such as football, wrestling, lacrosse and combative sports. The following localized movements of the cervical spine help improve flexibility, strength, and endurance of the musculature.

ANTERIOR SEMI-CIRCLES

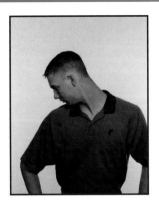 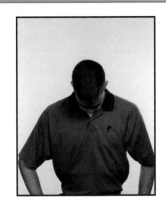 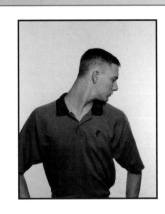

Introduction:
Full circumduction places unwarranted stress on cervical tendons and ligaments and is contraindicated in those with post trauma, disc problems, or post operative status. Anterior semi-circles are a general warming exercise initiated from a standing, sitting, or leaning position. A relaxed semi-circular motion is employed moving the head in pendular movements from side to side.

Method: Move head in half circles. Initiate movement by lowering head toward chest. Move chin towards top of one shoulder, then bring head back down to sternum (breast bone) and move it to opposite shoulder. Repeat sequence in opposite direction.

Repetitions: 8-10

HYPEREXTENSION

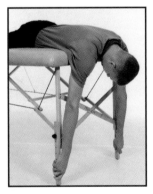 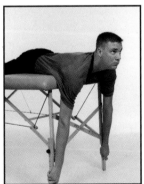

Muscles Stretched: Sternocleidomastoid and prevertebral muscles.

Muscles Strengthened: Upper erector spinae, splenius cervicis, splenius capitis, semispinalis cervicis and capitis.

Method: The exercise is performed in a four-point position on hands and knees or prone with the head extending beyond the edge of a table or bed. Initiate exercise by lowering head toward supportive surface and then extend head upward as far as possible without extending middle (thoracic) or lower (lumbar) spine.

Notes: Exercise should be performed slowly with gentle assisting stretch at end of movement. You may need assistance if doing the exercise on all fours.

Repetitions: 10 progressing to 15; more than one set may be beneficial.

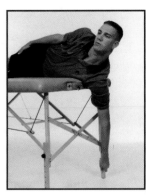

Muscles Strengthened: The three right scaleni — sternocleidomastoid, erector spinae and prevertebral muscles.

Muscles Stretched: The same muscles on the opposite side.

Method: Assume a side-lying position and then move head downward toward lower shoulder and upward toward top shoulder, giving a gentle stretch to muscles at that point.

Compensation Check: To help prevent lateral trunk flexion, hold onto table leg with full arm extension. Prevent levator scapula substitution (shrug) by placing top arm along thigh to help prevent shrugging of top shoulder. You can help prevent cervical rotation by looking at an object that is eye level.

Notes: Do not rotate or extend head backwards during the exercise.

Repetitions: Begin with 10 repetitions or a lesser number according to ability or previous history. Progress to 15 repetitions. More than one set may be desirable.

ROTATION: RIGHT

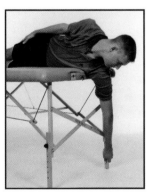
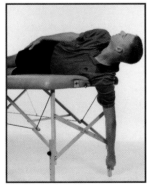

Muscles Strengthened: Right sternocleidomastoid, deep posterior spinal muscles, longissimus cervicis, splenius capitis and cervicis, and erector spinae.

Muscles Stretched: Counterparts on the opposite side.

Method: In a side-lying position, this exercise is performed from a downward, rotated position. Slowly rotate head upward and to the right. Stretch gently at top of motion. Release and return to starting position.

Compensation Check: Do not lateral flex trunk and rotate shoulder complex or allow top shoulder to shrug.

Repetitions: 10 if capable or a lesser number according to ability or previous history. Progress to 15 repetitions. More than one set may be desirable.

LATERAL FLEXION: LEFT

Muscles Strengthened: The three left scaleni — sternoclei-domastoid, erector spinae and prevertebral muscles.

Muscles Stretched: The opposite side (right) of the same group of muscles mentioned.

Method: Assume a side-lying position and then move head downward toward lower shoulder and upward toward top shoulder, giving a gentle stretch to muscles at that point.

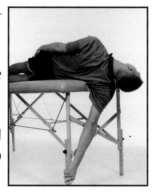 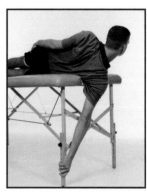

Compensation Check: To help prevent lateral trunk flexion, hold onto table leg with full arm extension. Prevent levator scapula substitution (shrug) by placing top arm along thigh to help prevent shrugging of top shoulder. You can help prevent cervical rotation by looking at an object that is eye level.

Notes: Do not rotate or extend head backwards during the exercise.

Repetitions: Begin with 10 repetitions or a lesser number according to ability or previous history. Progress to 15 repetitions. Two sets may be desirable.

ROTATION: LEFT

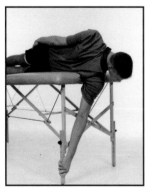 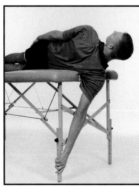

Muscles Strengthened: Left sternocleidomastoid, deep posterior spinal muscles, longissimus cervicis, splenius capitis and cervicis, and erector spinae.

Muscles Stretched: Counterparts on the opposite side.

Method: In a side lying position, this exercise is performed from a downward, rotated position. Slowly rotate head upward and to the left. Gently stretch at top of motion. Release and return to starting position.

Compensation Check: Do not lateral flex trunk and rotate shoulder complex or allow top shoulder to shrug.

Repetitions: 10 if capable or a lesser number according to ability or previous history. Progress to 15 repetitions. More than one set may be desirable.

Muscles Strengthened: Sternocleidomastoid and prevertebral muscles.

Muscles Stretched: Cervical erector spinae, splenius cervicis, splenius capitis, semispinalis cervicis, and semispinalis capitis muscles.

Method: Exercise is performed in a supine position. Retain shoulders on table throughout exercise. Tuck chin as close as possible to neck, lift head as far as possible in a close tuck. You may provide aid at any point throughout range or at end of movement with gentle assistance of your hand(s). Return to starting position and repeat.

Repetitions: 10 repetitions if capable or a lesser number according to ability or previous history. Progress to 15 repetitions. Two sets may be desirable.

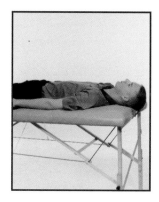 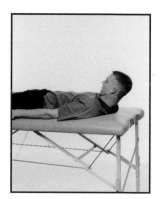 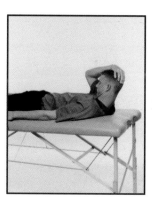

SHOULDER FLEXIBILITY

The following exercises are specifically designed to stretch glenohumeral, acromioclavicular, sternoclavicular and scapular musculature, and connective tissue. They are intended to help prevent muscle strains, joint sprains, and dislocations; help improve performance of the shoulder regions; and are beneficial postinjury and postsurgery. These flexibility exercises work every muscle fiber in the shoulders and should be done in the order presented for maximum results. They are best done standing, although they can be done sitting, providing there is room for arms to move freely.

CIRCUMDUCTION

Introduction: Circumduction increases circulation in the shoulder complex and arm. Perform arm circles toward and away from body mid line. Arms should hang like wet noodles when doing bent-over circumduction.

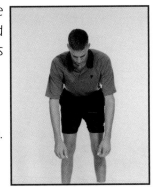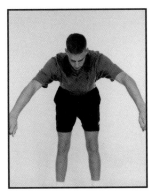

Method: Lean body forward, bend knees, and tighten stomach muscles. Begin with small circles and increase in size. You may also do giant arm circles (circumduction) from a standing position if shoulder is not sore or injured.

Repetitions: 10-15 in each direction.

HORIZONTAL ABDUCTION

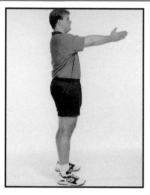 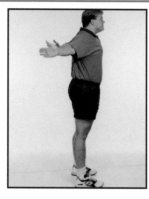 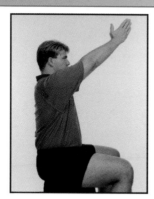 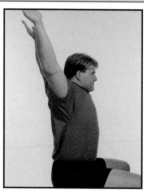

Muscles Stretched: Anterior chest and shoulder muscles including the pectoralis major, teres major and anterior deltoid by contracting the trapezius, rhomboid major and rhomboid minor muscles.

Method: Face palms forward with arms 8 to 12 inches below shoulder height. Reach backward, keeping arms straight, and draw shoulder blades (scapulae) as close together as possible. Return to starting position with palms together. Repeat exercise raising level of arms with each repetition in order to include the upper pectoral fibers.

Alternate Method: You may incorporate the use of a wall, doorway, or suitable stabilizing surface to assist with the stretch. To properly stretch these muscles, reach backward with the arm as the you rotate away from the stabilizing surface. Return to the starting position and repeat. Gradually elevate arms to lengthen the fibers above those previously stretched.

Repetitions: 10 or more if needed.

HYPEREXTENSION (OPEN AND WITH HANDS CLASPED)

Muscles Stretched: Biceps brachii and anterior deltoid muscles (plus the anterior serratus and lower pectorals).

Muscles Contracted: Triceps brachii and posterior deltoid muscles.

Method Part 1: Stand or sit erect, keep arms close to side, reach both arms back as far as possible. Release and return to starting position.

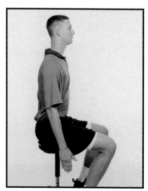 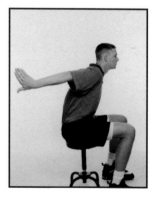

Repetitions: 6-8

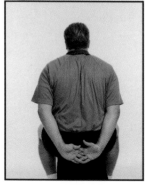 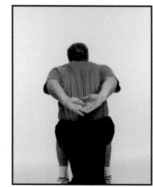

Method Part 2: Following this single arm shoulder hyperextension, clasp hands, palms facing away from body (which keeps shoulder blades apart) and keeping your elbows extended, reach back as far as possible without bending trunk forward or allowing shoulder blades to come together (adduct). Release and return to starting position.

Repetitions: 8-10

ROTATOR CUFF STRETCHES

The most frequent injury to the shoulder involves the rotator cuff muscles. Considerable attention must be given to the thorough stretching of this area. The important exercises include external rotation, internal rotation, horizontal flexion I, and horizontal flexion II.

EXTERNAL ROTATION

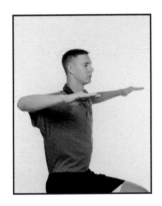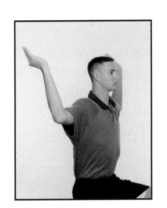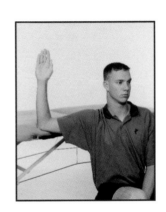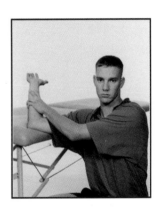

Muscles Stretched: Internal shoulder rotators including the teres major, subscapularis, latissimus dorsi, and pectoralis major muscles.

Muscles Contracted: Supraspinatus, infraspinatus and teres minor.

Method: Keeping arms (elbows) level with shoulders, bend elbows at 95-degree angle. The palms face downward as the exercise begins. Rotate shoulders (humerus) backward (externally) as far as possible by contracting the supraspinatus, infraspinatus, and teres minor muscles. Perform a slow steady stretch at end of the movement. Rest on a table or other support surface and assist with opposite hand.

Notes: A rope, bat, or handle may be gently used for aid with the opposite hand assisting. Lower to starting position and repeat.

Repetitions: 8-10

INTERNAL ROTATION

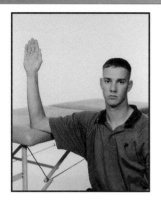 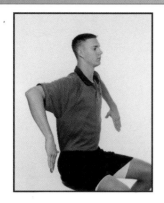 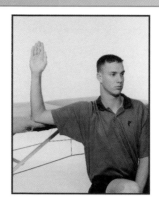 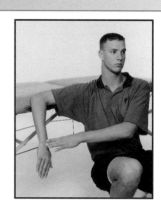

Muscles Contracted: Teres major, subscapularis and pectoralis major muscles.

Method: Bend elbows at 95-degree angle, level with shoulders, palms facing forward. Rotate shoulders (humerus) forward (internally) as far as possible by contracting the teres major, subscapularis, and pectoralis major muscles. Perform a slow steady stretch at end of each movement. You may support your elbow on table or other support surface and assist with opposite hand. Release and return to starting position and repeat.

Compensation Check: Keep scapula from compensating upward for best stretch of supraspinatus, infraspinatus, and teres minor.

Notes: Athletes are often limited in internal rotation sometimes resulting in rotary cuff injuries from throwing or from a severe blow or fall. In this case, you may need assistance to stabilize scapula to affect best maximum stretch. A rope, bat, or handle may also be used for aid with the opposite hand assisting.

Repetitions: 10-15

HORIZONTAL FLEXION I

Muscles Stretched: Rhomboid major, rhomboid minor, and external rotators, especially the teres minor and the infraspinatus.

Muscles Contracted: Pectoralis major, anterior deltoid, and coracobrachialis.

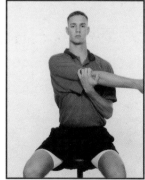

Method: Maintain straight elbow and keep shoulder parallel. Reach arm toward outside corner of opposite shoulder 3 to 4 inches below top of the shoulder, contracting pectoralis major, anterior deltoid, and coracobrachialis muscles.

Notes: Be sure exercising arm clears the top of the same side pectoral tissue; however, do not shrug shoulder or allow shoulder to move forward as straight arm reaches to touch opposite shoulder. Use opposite hand on elbow to assist with stretch at end of movement. Return arm to the side after each repetition.

Repetitions: 8-10

HORIZONTAL FLEXION II

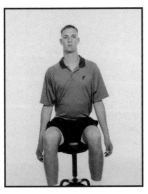 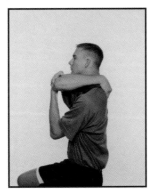

Muscles Stretched: Trapezius and rotator cuff, including supraspinatus, infraspinatus, and teres minor muscles.

Muscles Contracted: Pectoralis major, anterior deltoid, and coracobrachialis.

Method: Reach around to opposite side of neck. Contract pectoralis major, anterior deltoid, and coracobrachialis muscles. Walk the fingers down upper back as far as possible. Place free hand on elbow of exercising arm for gentle assistance at end of movement. Return the arm to side after each repetition.

Compensation Check: Do not allow exercising shoulder to shrug or move forward during this exercise.

Repetitions: 8-10

DELTOID STRETCH

Muscles Stretched: Middle and posterior deltoid fibers.

Muscles Contracted: Pectoralis major, subscapularis, and teres major.

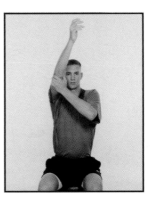 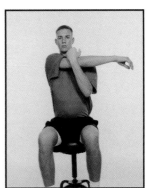

Method: Place arm in a vertical position with elbow extended and palm facing toward the body. Move the arm downward (diagonally) toward the front of opposite shoulder, contracting the pectoralis major, subscapularis, and teres major. During last few degrees of movement, rotate shoulder inward for maximum stretch. Use opposite hand to assist stretch effort. Move arm to vertical position after each stretch.

Notes: It is especially beneficial to stretch the supraspinatus muscle at the end of the movement by further lowering the arm beyond the breast bone.

Repetitions: 8-10

TRICEPS STRETCH

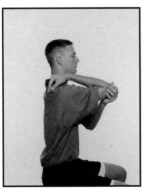 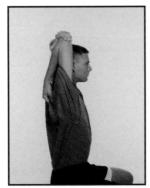

Muscles Stretched: Triceps brachii.

Muscles Contracted: Biceps brachii and anterior deltoid.

Method: Begin with elbow flexed 90 degrees forward from vertical position, palm facing toward mid line. With elbow flexed, contract biceps brachii and anterior deltoid muscles. Extend flexed arm upward as far as possible and assist stretch gently with opposite hand. Return to starting position after each repetition.

Repetitions: 6-10

FORWARD ELEVATION

Muscles Stretched: Upper triceps, posterior deltoid, and serratus anterior for greater upward movement of arm.

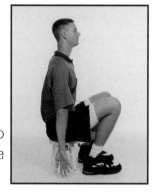
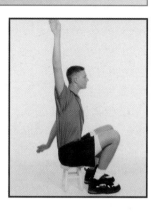

Muscles Contracted: Upper biceps brachii and anterior deltoid.

Introduction: Lack of full forward elevation contributes to many shoulder problems. The arm should be able to reach a complete vertical position without bending the elbow.

Method: From a sitting or standing position, reach one arm forward directly over top of shoulder as far as possible contracting the upper biceps brachii and anterior deltoid muscles. Keep palms facing body and elbows extended throughout movement. Counterbalance spinal extension (low back) compensation by contracting the abdominal muscles and reaching the opposite arm back as far as possible. You may alternate left and right arms. It may be necessary to stretch triceps first in order to achieve maximum forward elevation.

Compensation Check: Complete the exercise without rotating upper torso, arching back, or allowing elbows to bend.

Notes: You may use the top or side of a doorway to assist stretch. Reach arm upward while moving body forward to assist stretch.

Advanced Positions: An advanced exercise for athletes can be accomplished by internally rotating humerus (palm facing away from mid line) and performing the same basic forward elevation procedure.

Repetitions: 8-10

SIDEWARD ELEVATION

Muscles Stretched: Teres major, latissimus dorsi, sternal portion of the pectoralis major, and serratus muscles.

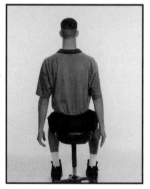
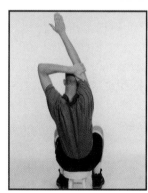

Muscles Contracted: Deltoids, trapezius, and rotator cuff muscles.

Introduction: This movement provides maximum upward rotation of the scapula, permitting maximum sideward elevation of shoulder complex.

Method: Face palm forward and keep elbow locked throughout movement. Reach upward as far as possible by contracting the deltoids, trapezius, and rotator cuff muscles while stretching the teres major, latissimus dorsi, sternal portion of the pectoralis major, and serratus muscles. Cross arm in back of head. Reach across mid line, assist with opposite hand, elbow locked throughout movement. Assist by clasping elbow with the opposite hand. Return to starting position after each repetition.

Continued On Following Page

SIDEWARD ELEVATION (CON'T.)

Notes: At the point of maximum scapular movement, lean trunk laterally in direction arm has been moving to best stretch latissimus dorsi. Moving obliquely forward from this end posture will insure better stretch of serratus posterior. Moving obliquely backward will stretch the serratus anterior.

Advanced Positions: Athletes may wish to additionally stretch the deltoid muscles by rotating the shoulder inward another 90 degrees, with the palm facing downward, elbow extended, and fingers pointed toward the mid line.

Repetitions: 10-15

POSTERIOR HAND CLASP (APLEY SCRATCH TEST)

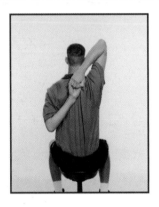 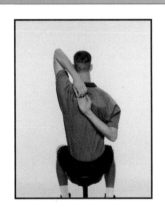 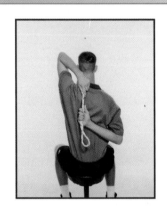 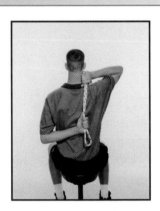

Muscles Stretched Upper Arm: Triceps, serratus anterior, and upper pectoral fibers.

Muscles Stretched Lower Arm: Long head of biceps brachii, supraspinatus, infraspinatus, and teres minor.

Method: Position the upper arm vertically against neck, palm facing body. As top arm reaches over (abduction) and downward (lateral rotation), the triceps, serratus anterior, and upper pectoral fibers are stretched. The opposite hand, palm facing away from body moves up spine between the shoulder blades attempting to clasp top hand. Join hands or move gently toward joining hands. As lower arm reaches under (medial rotation) and upward (adduction), the long head of biceps brachii, supraspinatus, infraspinatus, and teres minor are lengthened. At the end of the movement, you may assist an active effort with your free hand, assisting lower arm upward or top arm downward to increase both movements. Do not assist either movement unless active effort is sustained. Stretch gently to increase range.

Notes: It is not unusual that a person can do this well on one side but not on the other. For gentle assistance, use a rope or towel to help gain range needed to clasp hands. Each hand walks toward opposite hand. Work equally on the left and right side or you may experience greater risk of injuries when stressed in extended positions.

Repetitions: 8-10 each shoulder

ELBOW, RADIAL-ULNAR, WRIST, FINGER, AND THUMB FLEXIBILITY

Stretching may help reduce joint strain from weight bearing activities, sudden jolts, repeated stress from throwing, or torque, which may result in injuries such as Little League Elbow, Tennis Elbow, wrist or forearm strain. The elbows, wrists, and fingers are often neglected in sports preparation. The following stretches are helpful for increasing circulation and helping reduce joint and muscle stress or pain in the elbows, radial-ulnar, wrists, and hands.

ELBOW FLEXOR STRETCH

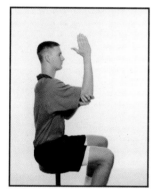 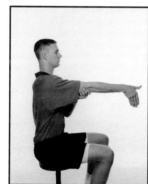

Muscles Stretched: Elbow flexors (biceps brachii, brachialis, brachioradialis).

Introduction: Stretching the elbow flexors helps insure maximum joint range and tissue extensibility to assist in reducing joint strain.

Method: Extend elbow with triceps brachii muscle to stretch biceps and brachialis muscles. With palm facing body mid line, ulnar flex wrist (little finger toward same side of wrist) to stretch brachioradialis muscle. Use free hand to stabilize elbow. Return to starting position and repeat.

Repetitions: 6-8

TRICEPS STRETCH

Muscles Stretched: Triceps brachii, a two-joint muscle of the posterior shoulder and elbow joints.

Muscles Contracted: Biceps brachii and anterior deltoid muscles.

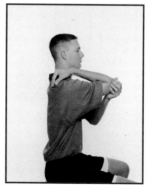 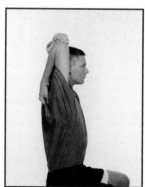

Method: Begin with elbow 90 degrees from vertical position with palm facing toward mid line. With elbow flexed, contract biceps brachii and anterior deltoid muscles. Extend flexed arm upward as far as possible and assist stretch gently with opposite hand. Return to starting position after each repetition.

Repetitions: 8-10

33

RADIAL-ULNAR PRONATION

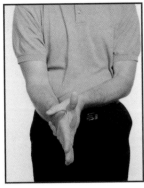 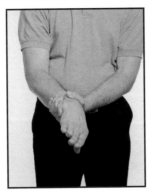 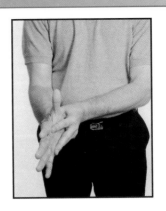 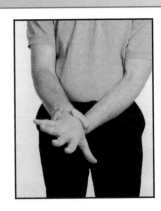

Muscles Stretched: Supinator and biceps brachii.

Muscles Contracted: Pronator quadratus and pronator teres.

Method: Flex elbow, adduct shoulder, and keep elbow against side of trunk throughout movement. From neutral position (thumb upward), rotate forearm inward to palm downward position. Clasp just below wrist with free hand for slight assisting stretch.

Alternate Technique: Place thumb, ring finger, and little finger around wrist and widely spread index finger and middle finger on palm of hand. Pronate hand with assistance of described hand. Release and repeat.

Notes: This exercise helps reduce elbow stress in movements causing torque, such as throwing, batting, and racket sports.

Repetitions: 6-8

RADIAL-ULNAR SUPINATION

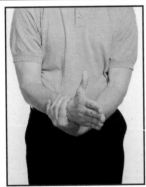 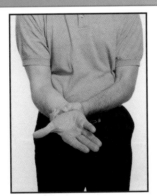 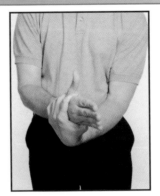 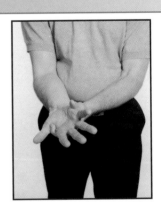

Muscles Stretched: Pronator quadratus and pronator teres.

Muscles Contracted: Supinator, biceps brachii and brachioradialis.

Method: Flex elbow 90 degrees, adduct shoulder, and maintain elbow against side of trunk throughout movement. From neutral position (thumb upward), rotate forearm outward moving palm upward, and pointing thumb downward while contracting the supinator, biceps brachii, and brachioradialis muscles. Clasp just below wrist and use free hand for slight assisting stretch.

Continued On Following Page

RADIAL-ULNAR SUPINATION (CON'T.)

Alternate Technique: Use assisting hand to clasp the exercising side with the middle finger, ring finger, and little finger below the wrist. Put the index finger around web between index finger and thumb, with the thumb approximately 2 inches below the base of index finger. Clasp firmly and assist. Release to starting position and repeat.

Notes: This stretch helps reduce elbow stress in throwing, batting, and racket sports.

Repetitions: 6-8

WRIST EXTENSION: PRONE

Muscles Stretched: Wrist and finger flexors, including the flexor carpi radialis, flexor carpi ulnaris, and flexor digitorums.

Muscles Contracted: Wrist and finger extensors including the extensor carpi radialis longus, extensor carpi radialis brevis, and extensor carpi ulnaris.

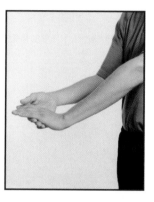 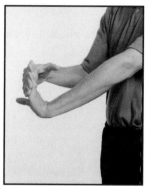

Method: Straighten elbow with palm facing downward. Extend wrist and fingers backward as far as possible by contracting wrist-finger extensors including the extensor carpi radialis longus, extensor carpi radialis brevis, extensor carpi ulnaris. For a gentle assisting stretch, use your free hand and finger muscles including the extensor digiti, extensor interosei, and extensor digitorum minimi. Place free hand over palmar surface of exercising hand covering base of fingers toward bottom of fingers surface. Make sure fingers continue to extend as free hand assists.

Notes: This exercise stretches wrist and finger flexors and helps reduce hand, wrist, forearm, and elbow stress.

Repetitions: 6-10

WRIST EXTENSION: SUPINE

Muscles Stretched: Wrist flexors at the proximal end attachments, including the flexor carpi radialis, flexor carpi ulnaris and flexor digitorums.

Muscles Contracted: Wrist-finger extensors including the extensor carpi radialis longus, extensor carpi radialis brevis, extensor carpi ulnaris, and extensor digitorum.

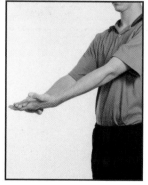 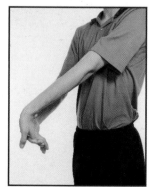

Continued On Following Page

Method: Lock elbow and face palm upward. Extend wrist and fingers back through full range by contracting wrist-finger extensors. Assist at end of movement with free hand by placing it over palmar surface of exercising hand, covering base of fingers toward top of fingers surface. Make sure fingers continue to extend as free hand assists.

Notes: This routine provides greater stretch of the wrist flexors and helps reduce hand, wrist, and forearm stress.

Repetitions: 6-10

WRIST FLEXION

Muscles Stretched: Wrist and forearm extensor muscles including the extensor carpi radialis longus, extensor carpi radialis brevis and extensor carpi ulnaris.

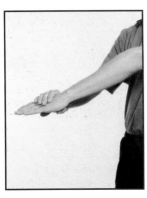
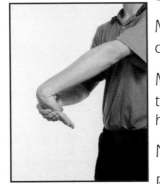

Muscles Contracted: Wrist flexor muscles including the flexor carpi radialis and flexor carpi ulnaris.

Method: Extend elbow. Slowly flex wrist downward by contracting wrist flexor muscles. Apply gentle stretch with opposite hand.

Notes: Helps reduce hand, wrist, forearm and elbow stress.

Repetitions: 6-8

FINGER EXTENSOR STRETCH

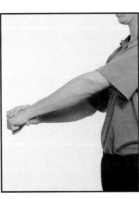
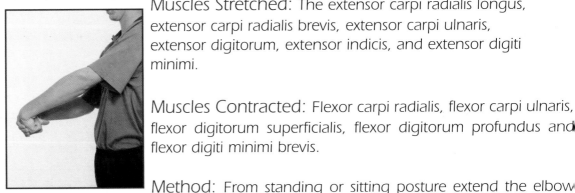

Muscles Stretched: The extensor carpi radialis longus, extensor carpi radialis brevis, extensor carpi ulnaris, extensor digitorum, extensor indicis, and extensor digiti minimi.

Muscles Contracted: Flexor carpi radialis, flexor carpi ulnaris, flexor digitorum superficialis, flexor digitorum profundus and flexor digiti minimi brevis.

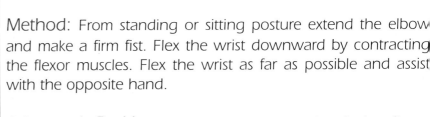

Method: From standing or sitting posture extend the elbow and make a firm fist. Flex the wrist downward by contracting the flexor muscles. Flex the wrist as far as possible and assist with the opposite hand.

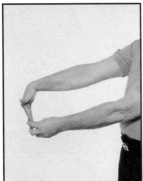
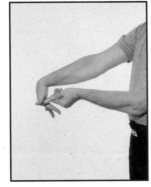

Advanced Positions: For maximal stretch of the finger extensor, flex wrist maximally, then flex individual finger as far as possible, and finally assist with opposite side thumb. Release to starting position and repeat.

Repetitions: 6-10

FINGER FLEXOR STRETCH

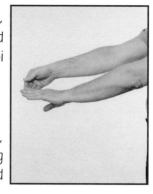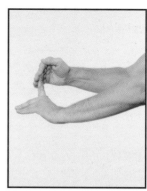

Muscles Stretched: Finger flexors including the lumbricales, flexor digitorum superficialis, flexor digitorum profundus, and flexor digiti minimi. The wrist flexors including the flexor carpi radialis and flexor carpi ulnaris also receive stretch.

Muscles Contracted: Working extensor muscles of the fingers including the extensor digiti minimi, extensor digitorum, and extensor indicis. Also the wrist extensor muscles including extensor carpi radialis longus, extensor carpi radialis brevis, and extensor carpi ulnaris.

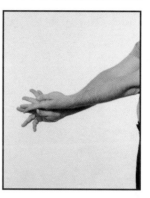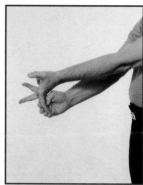

Method: Extend the wrist and fingers backward and assist with the opposite hand. Release and repeat. For best result, keep elbow extended. Perform exercise a number of repetitions from prone (palm down) position and then do same from supine (palm up) position.

Notes: The finest finger flexor stretch involves stretching one finger at a time. Extend finger far as possible and assist with opposite hand. For best results, place entire palm of hand along length of finger rather than only on the end of finger.

Repetitions: 6-10

FINGER-WRIST FLEXOR STRETCH

Muscles Stretched: Finger flexors including the flexor digitorum superficialis, flexor digitorum profundus and flexor digiti minimi. This stretch also involves the wrist flexor muscles including the flexor carpi radialis and flexor carpi ulnaris.

Muscles Contracted: Working extensor muscles of the fingers including the extensor digiti minimi, extensor digitorum, and extensor indicis. Also the wrist extensor muscles including extensor carpi radialis longus, extensor carpi radialis brevis, and extensor carpi ulnaris.

Method: From standing or sitting position, contract the working extensor muscles of the fingers. Also contract the wrist extensor muscles. Begin with palms facing away from body and flex the elbows 90 degrees. To stretch the finger-wrist flexors, hyperextend the wrist, and extend the fingers and elbows simultaneously. Release and repeat.

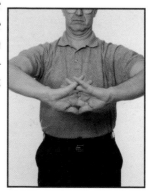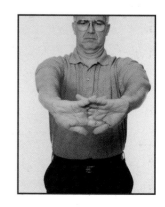

Repetitions: 6-10 repetitions.

FINGER ADDUCTOR (WEB) STRETCH

Muscles Stretched: The webs between each finger and the interossei palmaris muscles located between each finger.

Muscles Contracted: Interossei dorsalis and abductor digiti minimi muscles.

Method: Working with one finger at a time, abduct (spread) the finger by contracting the interossei dorsalis and abductor digiti minimi muscles. To assist the stretch use the thumb and an additional finger from the free hand. Stretch, release, and repeat.

Repetitions: 6-10

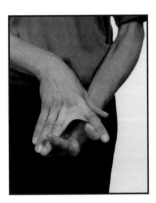

THUMB STRETCHING

The thumb is a comprehensive, versatile digit that is used countless times per day often with considerable stress. The thenar muscles at the flexor base of the thumb are used in most grasping activities. Four primary stretches of the thumb are described below.

THUMB OPPOSITION STRETCH

Introduction: Muscles that are involved in opposition include the opponens pollicis, flexor pollicis brevis and adductor pollicis muscles.

Method: Placing your hand with the palm facing away from the body and your thumb at 90-degree angle to index finger, horizontally abduct the thumb away from the index finger, using the extensor pollicis longus and extensor pollicis brevis. Move the thumb back toward the body. Use your opposite hand to assist as if you are drawing back on a bowstring. Release and repeat.

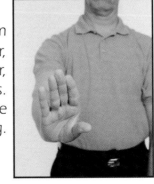 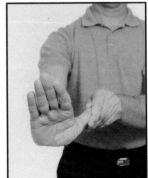

Repetitions: 6-8

THUMB ADDUCTOR (WEB) STRETCH

Introduction: The adductor pollicis longus and adductor pollicis brevis move the thumb inward toward the index finger forming an inward pinching motion. The web is also contained there.

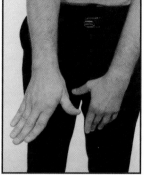 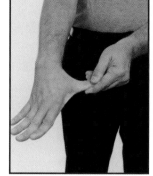

Method: Abduct the thumb horizontally moving the thumb laterally away from the index finger. Contracting the abductor pollicis longus and abductor pollicis brevis, stretch the web and adductors using the opposite hand to assist. Release and repeat.

Repetitions: 6-8

THUMB ABDUCTOR STRETCH

Introduction: The thumb muscles, the abductor pollicis longus and abductor pollicis brevis, which move the thumb away from (abduction) the index finger are seldom stretched.

Method: Contracting the adductor pollicis longus and adductor pollicis brevis, actively move the thumb over the top of the neighboring index finger. Use the opposite hand to assist the stretch. Release and repeat.

Repetitions: 6-8

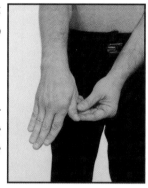 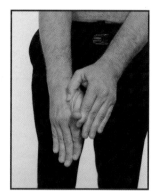

THUMB EXTENSOR STRETCH

Introduction: Muscles that extend the thumb include the extensor pollicis longus and extensor pollicis brevis.

Method: Contracting the opponens pollicis, flexor pollicis brevis, and adductor pollicis, actively contract the muscles of opposition by moving the thumb towards the base of the little finger. Use your free (opposite) hand by placing the thumb on outer base of thumb being stretched. Flex toward little finger. Release and repeat.

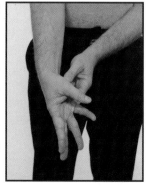 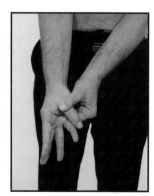

Repetitions: 6-8

HIP FLEXIBILITY

The muscles of the hip joint are among the most frequently injured. Many of the muscles that flex and extend the hip are also part of the low back and knee. Inflexibility of these joint muscles can limit hip, pelvic girdle, and low back movements. Hip inflexibility also limits walking and running stride and gait, lateral movements, and quickness.

BENT KNEE HAMSTRING STRETCH

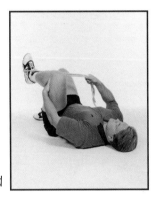 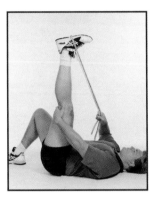 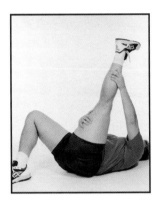

Muscles Stretched: Especially good stretch for distal lower hamstrings (area above insertion).

Method: From a supine position, place one hand under or in front of active knee to help maintain flexed hip. Flex uninvolved leg, especially if back is a problem. Contract quadriceps, extend knee of leg to be stretched slowly to full extension. Do not flex hip additionally unless knee can extend completely. Gradually flex hip (which moves active leg toward head). You will be able to move leg farther as lower hamstring flexibility improves. As quadriceps muscles continue to move leg, gently assist with a rope or your free hand. Release to starting position and repeat.

Repetitions: Two sets of 10, alternating legs after each set.

BENT KNEE "INNER HAMSTRING STRETCH"

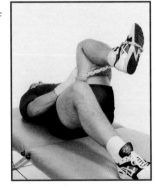 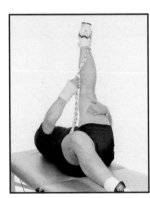

Muscles Stretched: Provides greater isolation for insertion of semitendinosus and semimembranosus muscles (distal end).

Method: Rotate lower part of leg (tibia) outward while performing previously described Bent Knee Hamstring Stretch. Place rope under foot and wrap both strands of rope around outside of ankle. Do not allow upper leg (femur) to turn as lower leg rotates. Extend knee, moving lower leg toward same side shoulder. Use rope to assist at point of stretch. Release and repeat.

Repetitions: One or two sets of 10.

BENT KNEE "OUTER HAMSTRING STRETCH"

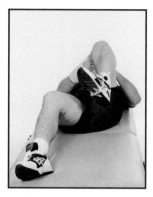
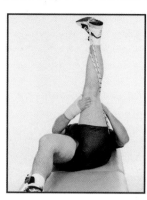

Muscles Stretched: Provides greater isolation of distal insertions of biceps femoris muscle.

Method: Rotate lower part of leg (tibia) inward (medial) while performing previously described Bent Knee Hamstring Stretch. Place rope under foot and wrap both strands around inside of ankle. Do not allow upper leg (femur) to turn as lower leg rotates. Extend knee, moving lower leg toward same side shoulder. Assist by using free hand with rope. Stretch, release, and repeat.

Notes: The biceps femoris is a frequently pulled muscle having two insertions heads, one inserting below the knee.

Repetitions: One or two sets of 10.

HAMSTRING STRETCH: BENT KNEE SEATED

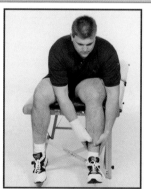
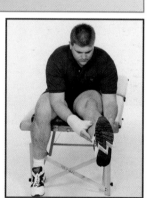

Muscles Stretched: Isolation of the distal insertion of the hamstrings.

Introduction: This is a good stretch for athletic persons with tight lower hamstrings who are free of back problems.

Method: From a seated position, lean body forward, contract abdominal muscles and lift leg with quadriceps. Use hands to provide gentle assistance at end of movement, release and repeat. Lean trunk farther forward as flexibility increases.

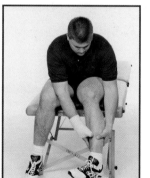
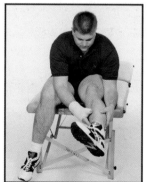

Notes: Eventually, athlete should be able to touch chest on knees and lock knee in extension.

Advanced Positions: Rotate lower part of leg inward to isolate insertion end of biceps femoris. Rotate lower part of leg outward to isolate insertion ends of semitendinosus and semimembranosus muscles.

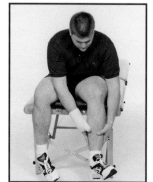
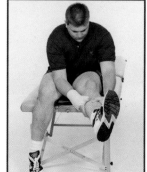

Repetitions: Two or three sets of 10 for each leg depending on range limitation.

STRAIGHT LEG HAMSTRING STRETCH

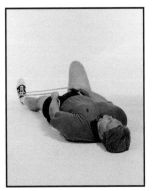 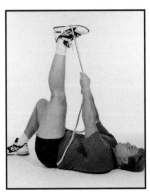 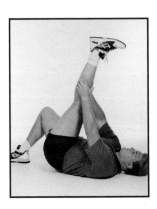

Muscles Stretched: Proximal hamstring muscles.

Muscles Contracted: Quadriceps muscles.

Method: From a supine position, slowly lift one leg using the quadriceps muscles. Give gentle assistance with rope or hands at end of movement as quadriceps muscles continue to move leg. If using a rope, walk hands up rope, hand over hand, as you lift leg upward. Release to starting position and repeat.

Notes: Flex nonexercising leg 25 to 50 degrees especially if there is a severe back consideration. Nonexercising leg may remain on the surface if hamstrings are quite flexible.

Compensation Check: Do not allow exercising leg to bend at any point in movement.

Repetitions: Two sets of 10, alternating legs after each set.

STRAIGHT LEG "INNER HAMSTRING STRETCH"

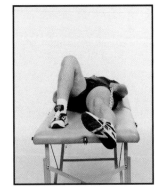 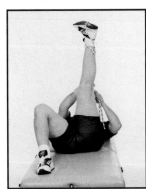

Muscles Stretched: Medial hamstring muscles — semitendinosus and semimembranosus.
Following the straight leg hamstring stretch the medial hamstring muscles may require greater isolated stretching.

Method: From the same position as the Straight Leg Hamstring Stretch, isolate the proximal medial hamstrings by rotating the leg (femur) inward. Place the rope under foot with both strands around inside of lower part of leg to help maintain leg in an internal rotated position. Lock knee by contracting front leg (quadriceps) muscles and lift with hip abductors (outer thigh) and quadriceps. Walk hands up the rope. Release and repeat.

Repetitions: One or two sets of 10.

STRAIGHT LEG "OUTER HAMSTRING STRETCH"

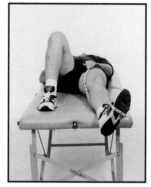 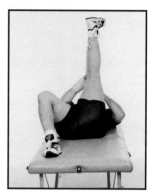

Muscles Stretched: Outer hamstring (biceps femoris).

Muscles Contracted: Hip adductors and quadriceps.

Method: From same position as Straight Leg Hamstring Stretch, keep knee extended (quadriceps contracted) and rotate entire leg outward. Move leg toward opposite side shoulder by contracting hip adductors (inner thigh). Place rope under foot then loop both strands around outside of lower leg to help maintain the leg in an outward rotated position. Nonexercising leg is internally rotated and adducted well beyond midline of opposite side leg. For best results, place rope in opposite side hand or use both hands to walk up rope, as leg reaches toward opposite side shoulder.

Notes: The biceps femoris is a frequently pulled muscle having two insertions heads, one inserting below the knee. The tensor fascia latae, gluteus maximus, piriformis and other lateral thigh muscles should first be stretched to assure maximal stretch with least compensation and interference. (See the following exercises for stretching these muscles: Hip External Rotator, Hip Internal Rotator, Hip Abductor, Hip Flexion, Lateral Gluteus Maximus, and Piriformis.)

Repetitions: Two sets of 10, alternating legs after each set.

HAMSTRING STRETCH: STRAIGHT LEGS, SEATED

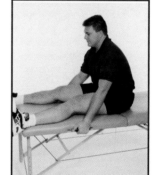 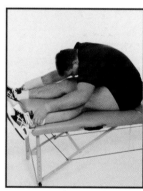

Muscles Stretched: Hamstrings.

Muscles Contracted: Quadriceps.

Introduction: This is an advanced exercise for those who are very flexible or for those athletes, such as gymnasts or swimmers, who require extreme flexibility in their sport.

Method: Starting from a seated position with legs out straight, tuck the chin, exhale, firmly tighten the abdominals, and lean forward. Contract quadriceps to keep knees from bending. Do exercise slowly without bouncing. Use hands for light assisted stretch at end of movement. Resume sitting position and repeat.

Notes: It is safest to do this after stretching hamstrings and long back muscles. Do not do this exercise if you have pain or disc involvement of the back.

Repetitions: 10.

HAMSTRING STRETCH: STANDING

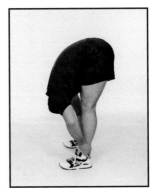

Muscles Stretched: Hamstrings

Muscles Contracted: Quadriceps and abdominals.

Method: From a standing position, contract the abdominal muscles, so that the back muscles may be stretched passively without tension, and contract the quadriceps muscles (front thigh). Lean forward as far as possible to stretch hamstrings and low back. Release tension on back by slowly returning to the starting stance. Do movement slowly without bouncing. Use hands for gentle assisted stretch. Proximal and lower ends of hamstrings and lower back should be stretched prior to this exercise.

Notes: This stretch is best used after body is really warmed up and between competitive movements when you feel a tightness in the hamstrings and back.

Repetitions: 8-10.

PSOAS STRETCH: PRONE

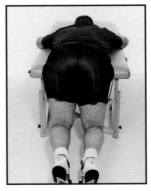
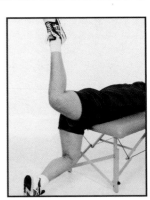
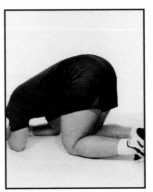
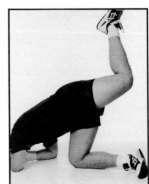

Muscles Stretched: Psoas and iliacus muscles.

Muscles Contracted: Hip extensors (gluteus maximus and hamstrings).

Method: Rest upper body and pelvis on table with no weight on contralateral (nonactive) leg. Keep nonactive leg against table. Flex exercising leg 90 degrees at knee and keep leg adducted against nonexercising thigh throughout movement. Extend hip, stretching psoas at end of movement. Stretch and release to starting position.

Notes: The same exercise may be accomplished on the floor in a three-point position.

Repetitions: 10.

PSOAS STRETCH: SIDE LYING

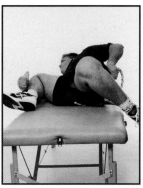

Muscles Stretched: Psoas.

Muscles Contracted: Gluteus maximus (buttocks) and upper hamstrings.

Method: From a side-lying position, move lower, uninvolved, leg close to chest and secure with lower arm. Hand may be placed under thigh or under bottom of foot for stability. Maintain top hip in vertical position and thigh close to lower thigh throughout movement. Place rope around top ankle. Maintain knee at 95 to 100 degree angle. Contract gluteus maximus (buttock) and upper hamstrings of top leg reaching straight backward using rope to assist at end of movement. Return to starting position and repeat.

Repetitions: One or two sets of 10.

PSOAS STRETCH: KNEELING

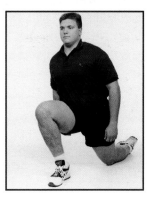

Muscles Stretched: Psoas and iliopsoas.

Muscles Contracted: Gluteus maximus (buttock) and upper hamstrings.

Method: From a three-point kneeling position, begin with weight on knee of leg to be stretched. Moving forward onto flexed front leg, keep top of pelvis tilted backward throughout movement by contracting stomach muscles. As you move forward, contract gluteus maximus (buttock) and upper hamstring muscles. Maintain body in a vertical position to stretch iliopsoas muscles. Release and repeat.

Repetitions: 10-15.

PSOAS STRETCH: SUPINE

Muscles Stretched: Psoas.

Muscles Contracted: Gluteus maximus (buttock) and upper hamstrings.

Method: Lying on your back (supine), flex the nonactive leg to your chest to help prevent compensation by extending the lower back. Stabilize with the same side hand if necessary. Contract the abdominals to help prevent back extension. Place rope around opposite side ankle. Keep knee at 95 to 100 degree angle and using buttock (gluteus maximus) and upper hamstrings, extend hip backward and assist with rope.

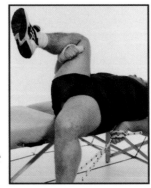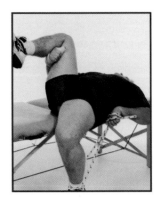

Repetitions: One or two sets of 10.

RECTUS FEMORIS STRETCH: SIDE LYING

Muscles Stretched: Rectus femoris (quadriceps) muscle(s).

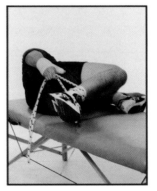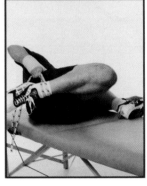

Method Part 1: Lie on one side with lower hip flexed and thigh pulled close to your chest. This prevents back extension. Maintain position by using same side hand for stabilization. Hand may be placed under foot of stabilized leg or around thigh if you are unable to clasp foot. Contract abdominal muscles to help prevent forward tilt of pelvis. Maintain upper leg in adduction position toward body midline throughout movement and do not point knee to far upward. To stretch hip flexor (proximal) end of rectus femoris, extend thigh back to near straight line with upper body. Flex knee, with heel toward buttock using hamstrings. Assist with rope. Release.

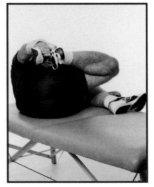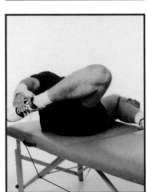

Repetitions: 10-15 to release upper thigh (hip flexor end).

Method Part 2: To stretch lower end of rectus femoris, flex top leg and grasp ankle with hand. Contract gluteus maximus and hamstrings reaching backward with thigh. Use hand for gentle assistance at end of movement. Repeat.

Caution: If you have extremely short rectus femoris muscles, it may be necessary to decrease flexion of top leg and use rope to assist.

Repetitions: Two sets of 10 alternating legs.

RECTUS FEMORIS STRETCH: STANDING

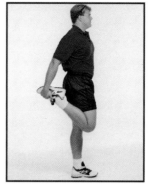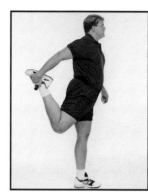

Introduction: When you have limited time between periods of play or athletic activity, and if you have already adequately stretched the quadriceps, you may stretch quadriceps and hip flexors from standing position.

Method: Tighten abdominals to prevent back from arching. Exercising thigh should be kept adducted and tight against opposite thigh. Extending thigh backward, contract gluteus maximus and hamstrings. Provide gentle assistance with hand at end of movement.

Repetitions: 10 each leg.

HIP EXTERNAL ROTATOR STRETCH: PRONE

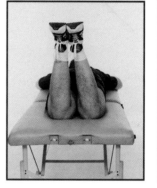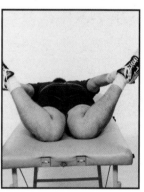

Muscles Stretched: External rotators of the hip (six deep external rotators and gluteus maximus).

Muscles Contracted: Internal hip rotators (gluteus minimus, tensor fascia latae).

Introduction: The ability to move laterally, pivot, or change directions may be limited by the inflexibility or lack of strength of the hip rotators.

Method: In a prone position (lying on your stomach) with knees together, rotate hips inward moving lower legs laterally away from midline as far as possible. As your muscles loosen at that angle moves knees farther apart. Continue moving farther apart until each external rotator has been stretched. Use hands for assistance at end of movement. Keep hips flat on surface.

Repetitions: 10-15.

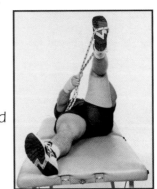
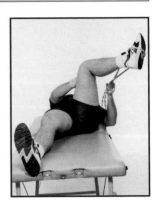

Muscles Stretched: The six deep external rotators (quadratus femoris, obturator externus, inferior gemellus, obturator internus, superior gemellus and piriformis muscles) and outer gluteus maximus.

Muscles Contracted: Gluteus medius, gluteus minimus, and tensor fascia latae.

Method: In a supine position (on your back), place a rope around midfoot — bending the knee at a right angle — and clasp the rope with the same side hand. Place the opposite hand on the knee to stabilize femur. Rotate hip by moving lower part of leg away from midline and assist at end of movement by using rope and continued muscle effort. To isolate each external rotator individually, move the thigh an additional 10 degrees away from midline from previous position.

Compensation Check: To prevent compensation of pelvis, which will attempt to hike in direction of lower leg movement, spread nonexercising leg away from the midline and turn it outward.

Notes: This stretch improves movement and restores range of motion.

Repetitions: One or two sets of 10.

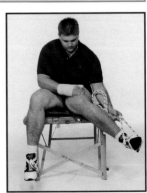

Muscles Stretched: The six deep external rotators and gluteus maximus.

Muscles Contracted: Gluteus minimus, gluteus medius, tensor fascia latae.

Introduction: Rotation improves the ability for lateral movement and increases the ability to change direction quickly. From a seated location, place a pad under the knees and loop a rope under your midfoot. Keeping your buttocks on the table, move the lower part of your leg away from midline without hiking same side of pelvis. Assist active movement with gentle assistance of rope. Move thigh farther away from midline as each rotator muscle is released. Move thigh until full limit has been reached. Release to neutral position and repeat.

Repetitions: 10-15.

HIP EXTERNAL ROTATOR STRETCH WITH HAND: SEATED

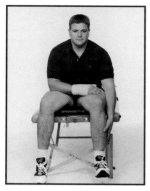 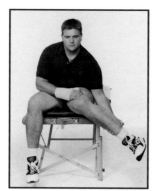

Muscles Stretched: Six deep external rotators and gluteus maximus.

Muscles Contracted: Internal rotators including gluteus minimus, gluteus medius, and tensor fascia latae.

Introduction: This is a good stretch (rotation) for warm-ups. It also increases lateral quickness and helps prevent injuries.

Method: Following the instructions for the previous exercise, remember to keep buttocks flat on surface. Move lower part of your leg away from midline without hiking the same side of the pelvis. Use hands to assist end of movement. Release to starting position and repeat.

Notes: If you have back problems, perform this exercise in a supine (lying) position as explained above.

Repetitions: 10-15.

HIP INTERNAL ROTATOR STRETCH: PRONE

Muscles Stretched: Internal rotators; tensor fascia latae and gluteus minimus, gluteus medius.

Muscles Contracted: Six deep external rotators and gluteus maximus.

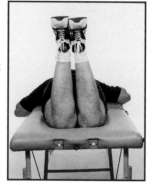 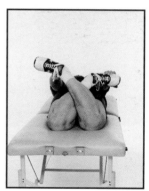

Method: From a prone position, move nonexercising leg far enough apart (about six inches) to allow full clearance of exercising leg. Keep hips flat on surface. Internally rotate active leg as far as possible by contracting medial rotators. Use opposite hand to assist stretch at end of movement. Stretch leg one at a time or simultaneously.

Repetitions: 10-15 each side.

HIP INTERNAL ROTATOR STRETCH WITH ROPE: SEATED

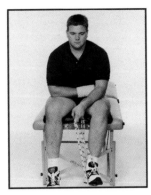 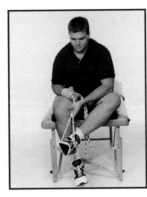

Muscles Stretched: Gluteus minimus, gluteus medius, and tensor fascia latae.

Muscles Contracted: Gluteus maximus and six deep external rotators.

Introduction: Helps to assist in developing quickness and in improving lateral movement.

Method: Placing a pad under knees, assume a seated position. Using a rope looped under the midfoot, move your leg across midline as far as possible while keeping opposite side buttock flat on table. Prevent opposite side of the pelvis from lifting. Use the rope to assist at end of the active effort. Return to neutral position and repeat.

Repetitions: 10-15.

HIP INTERNAL ROTATOR STRETCH WITH HAND: SEATED

Muscles Stretched: Gluteus minimus, gluteus medius, tensor fascia latae.

Muscles Contracted: Gluteus maximus and six deep external rotators.

Introduction: This excellent warm-up can also be done on floor or field to help maximize change of direction and speed for many sports.

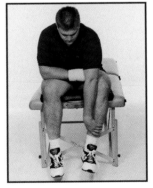 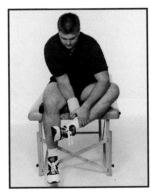

Method: In seated position similar to that described in the previous exercise, move leg across midline. Do not hike opposite side of the pelvis. Use hands to assist end of movement. Release to starting position and repeat. To perform this exercise on the floor or playing field, stretch out the nonexercising leg and cross the ankle of the active leg over it. Do the exercise as indicated.

Notes: For relief of lower back problems, perform this exercise in a supine position (see following exercise) to keep pelvis flat or consult the assisted section.

Repetitions: 10-15.

HIP INTERNAL ROTATOR STRETCH: SUPINE

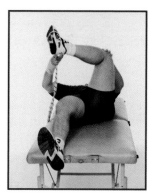

Muscles Stretched: Gluteus medius, gluteus minimus, and tensor fascia latae.

Muscles Contracted: Gluteus maximus and six deep external rotators.

Method: From a supine (on your back) position, flex knee at a 90-degree angle and place a rope around midfoot, clasping rope with opposite hand. Use the same side hand to stabilize the femur by gently clasping near knee. Rotate your hip by moving lower part of leg towards midline. Assist at end of range with rope and with continued muscle effort.

Compensation Check: Prevent compensation of pelvis, which will attempt to hike in direction of lower leg, by moving noninvolved leg across midline and rotating same leg inward.

Repetitions: One or two sets of 10.

HIP ABDUCTOR STRETCH

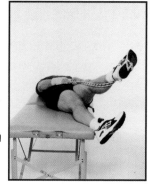 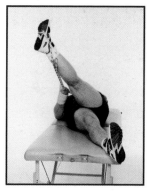

Muscles Stretched: Gluteus medius, vastus lateralis, tensor fascia latae, and iliotibial band.

Muscles Contracted: Anterior thigh muscles (quadriceps); pectinius; gracilis; and adductor(s) magnus, longus and brevis.

Introduction: When the muscles of the lateral hip and thigh are tight they may cause problems related to the back, the hips, or the knees.

Method: From a supine position, move nonexercising leg below exercising leg into hyperadduction beyond the midline and rotate entire nonactive leg inward. This combination of medial rotation and hyperadduction helps maintain pelvis in stable position throughout stretch movement. Place rope under bottom of foot and then wrap around lateral aspect of lower leg to provide assistance and help prevent compensation by medial rotation of femur and tibia. To do the exercise, keep the knee straight and externally rotate the leg (femur) 20 degrees. This is accomplished by contracting the anterior thigh muscles (quadriceps) throughout the movement. Contract pectinius; gracilis; and adductor(s) magnus, longus and brevis, and hyperadduct the extended thigh across midline as far as possible without internally rotating leg. Assist active movement by walking the hands up the rope. Release to starting position.

Notes: To stretch these muscles, the knee must remain completely straight.

Repetitions: One or two sets of 10.

51

HIP ADDUCTOR STRETCH (GROIN)

Muscles Stretched: Hip adductors, the gracilis, pectinius, adductor magnus, adductor longus and adductor brevis.

Muscles Contracted: Hip abductor muscles, gluteus medius, tensor fascia latae, and sartorius.

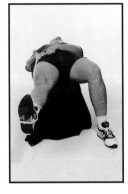 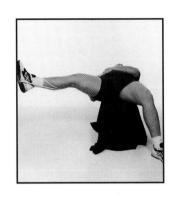

Method: Assume a supine position. Move the nonexercising leg far out as possible and rotate it outward. Internally rotate the active leg, keeping the leg straight. Use the rope looped over the foot on the outside of the heel and around to the inside of the ankle to help prevent external rotation of hip during abduction. (See photograph.) Perform exercise with foot pointed outward as far as possible. Contract anterior thigh (quadriceps) throughout movement. Move the exercising leg as far as possible and return to starting position. Use the rope for guidance and walk hands up rope to assist stretch at end of movement.

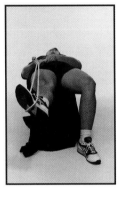 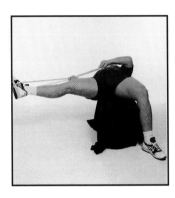

Repetitions: One or two sets of 10.

Additional Stretches: Following these sets, repeat the exercise with the active leg (femur) rotated outward 45 degrees to isolate adductor magnus more completely. Abduct and extend hip downward away from midline. To best isolate the adductor magnus, release internal rotation of rope. Externally rotate the leg 45 degrees simultaneously extending the thigh downward. Return to midline after each repetition and repeat.

Repetitions: One or two sets of 10.

HIP ADDUCTOR STRETCH (GROIN): SEATED

Muscles Stretched: Hip adductors — gracilis, pectinius, adductor magnus, adductor longus and adductor brevis.

Muscles Contracted: Hip abductors — gluteus medius, gluteus minimus, tensor fascia latae, and sartorius.

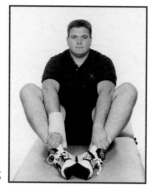 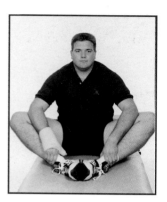

Method: Assume a seated position with the soles of feet placed together. Contract outside of hip, spreading thighs as far as possible. Return to adducted position and repeat. As you become more flexible move heels closer to the buttocks. Use hands to gently assist stretch at end of movement.

Notes: It is more difficult and less exacting to stretch the adductors from this position because of the forward tilt of the pelvis and because the femur externally rotates during abduction. In addition, the adductors are required to stabilize the pelvis and femur, which causes the adductors to eccentrically contract in order to achieve stabilization.

Repetitions: One or two sets of 10.

HIP FLEXION

Muscles Stretched: Gluteus maximus (buttock) and proximal end of hamstrings.

Muscles Contracted: Psoas, iliacus, and proximal rectus femoris muscles.

Introduction: This exercise improves the ability of the hip to flex and stretch the gluteus maximus and proximal end of hamstrings.

Method: From a supine position, bend the knee toward the same side axilla (arm pit). You may either keep the inactive leg straight or slightly flex it to prevent discomfort to back. Use your hands behind the thigh to prevent pressure on the knee and provide assistance at the end of active movement. Lower leg to starting position after each repetition.

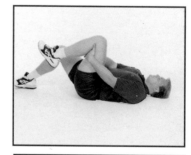

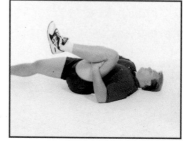

Notes: This exercise also may be performed in standing position.

Repetitions: One or two sets of 10.

LATERAL GLUTEUS MAXIMUS STRETCH

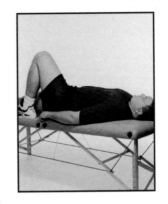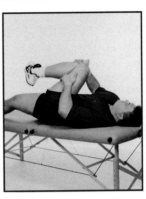

Muscles Stretched: Lower back rotators, outer hip, and especially the gluteus maximus.

Muscles Contracted: Hip flexors, abdominals, medial hip rotators, and hip adductors.

Introduction: This gentle stretch is ideal for lower back.

Method: From a supine position, stabilize your pelvis by moving nonexercising leg across midline and rotate same leg to inward extreme. A pad and seat belt may be used to help stabilize pelvis. Contract hip flexors abdominals, medial hip rotators, and hip adductors as you move the exercising leg towards bottom of opposite side breast. Use both hands on outside of knee to assist. Return to starting position and repeat.

Repetitions: One or two sets of 10.

PIRIFORMIS: FIGURE 4 ROTATOR STRETCH

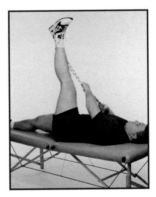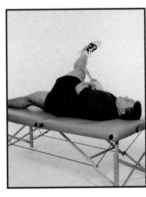

Muscles Stretched: Low back rotators, external hip rotators, and gluteus maximus muscles. (This is an especially good stretch for piriformis muscle.)

Method: From supine position, rotate nonexercising leg inward and move across midline (hyperadduct) as far as possible to help stabilize pelvis and isolate muscles to be stretched. Stretch opposite side muscles by extending knee to within 5 degrees of full extension and lifting leg upward to as near vertical as possible. Contract lower abdominals, internal hip rotators, and hip adductor muscles and reach across body as far as possible with scapulae (shoulder blades) and pelvic girdle remaining in contact with surface. A pad and seatbelt may be placed across pelvis for greater stabilization. Assist stretch movement with opposite side hand or by walking hands up a rope that has been looped around the mid foot and ankle. Return to starting position and gently repeat.

Repetitions: One or two sets of 10.

Notes: A partially flexed exercising side knee will help prevent biceps femoris (quad) and tensor fascia latae interference. This is an important stretch for those who wish to improve quickness and lateral movement and help relieve sciatic nerve radiation. See Assisted Hip: Figure 4 Rotator Stretch for how to assist those with back histories, pelvic distortions, or sciatic nerve involvement.

TRUNK FLEXIBILITY

The spine allows movement in all planes, and although the potential is there most of us do not utilize our maximum strength and range of motion in this area. To prevent injury and develop maximum power and quickness in a variety of sports and physical activities, this potential should be explored and reached. Limited flexion, extension, and rotation of the thoracic and lumbar (low back) spinal tissues may lead to injuries such as muscle pulls or low back problems. When properly stretched, muscles of the trunk and hip allow for freer pelvic movement. The following exercises address these issues, but please note that restoration of trunk flexibility following an injury or surgery should be done carefully.

SINGLE LEG PELVIC TILT

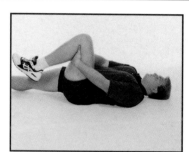

Muscles Stretched: This Williams Back Exercise helps attain maximum sacrospinalis (low back) and gluteus maximus flexibility.

Muscles Contracted: Hip flexor and abdominal muscles.

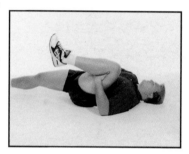

Caution: If condition is post operative, there is disc involvement, or there is severe pain, flex the nonexercising knee 25 or more degrees. Otherwise, the nonexercising knee may remain straight and in contact with the surface.

Method: From a supine position, flex the exercising knee and pull it toward the axilla (arm pit) by contraction of the hip flexor and abdominal muscles. Place the hands behind the thigh to prevent pressure on the knee and provide slight assistance at the end of free movement. Return thigh to vertical position and repeat.

Notes: If there is no major back condition, this exercise may be done in standing position.

Repetitions: 10 each side.

DOUBLE LEG PELVIC TILT

Muscles Stretched: Gluteus maximus and sacrospinalis (low back) muscles.

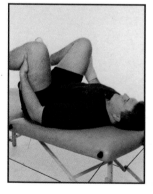
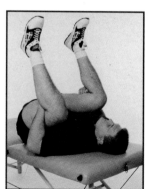

Method: Begin with knees and hips flexed at a 90-degree angle, thighs pointed vertical. Exhale and contract hip flexor and abdominal muscles, pulling the thighs toward the axilla (arm pits). Place hands under the thighs and assist the contracting muscles in the stretching movement. Return to the starting position (thighs vertical) and attempt to move closer to the axilla (armpit) with each repetition.

Repetitions: 10.

REVERSE CURL

Muscles Stretched: Thoracic and lumbar extensor muscles.

Muscles Contracted: Lower abdominal and hip flexor muscles.

Method: This stretch is accomplished by flexing the knees and lifting the pelvis. Contract the lower abdominal and hip flexor muscles, lifting until shoulder blades touch surface, then immediately lower slowly until feet touch surface again.

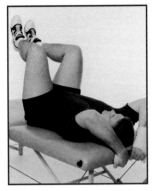 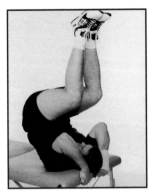

Contraindications: Extension of the legs over the head until the toes are touching the floor in back of the head is contraindicated because the back muscles are placed in a state of contraction (lengthening) while stretch is attempted. This position also puts extreme pressure on the neck.

Repetitions: 8-10.

TRUNK EXTENSION

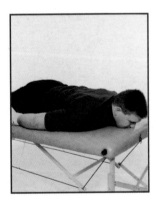 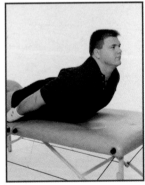

Muscles Stretched: Increases lumbar spine extension and flexibility of abdominal muscles including rectus abdominus, external obliques, internal obliques.

Muscles Contracted: Erector spinae muscles.

Method: In a prone position with lower body stabilized, contract erector spinae muscles (entire long back muscles) and lift head and shoulders while lower body remains on the surface. Use hands to assist extensor muscles at end of range. Lower body immediately after reaching extension. Repeat.

Contraindications: Extending the upper and lower body simultaneously is a dangerous, contraindicated exercise (rocker or banana) and may result in muscle spasm or low back injury.

*Caution: Trunk extension may initially be contraindicated for those with back histories.

Repetitions: 8-10.

THORACIC EXTENSION

Introduction: This stretch is especially helpful for the dorsal (anterior) thoracic spine and for those suffering from thoracic kyphosis (forward curvature).

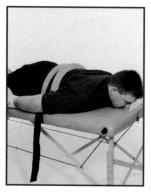 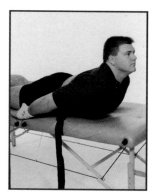

Method: From a prone position, stabilize the lower region of the thoracic spine by placing a pad and strap across that area or by asking someone to apply firm pressure to that area in a forward and downward direction. (For a better understanding of assisting with this exercise see Thoracic Extension: Assisted.) Once comfortably stabilized, extend upper back and neck.

Advanced Positions: Once you master this exercise, you may wish to add sandbag resistance to increase thoracic strength.

Repetitions: 8-10 or, for more serious problems, two or three series of 10 repetitions.

UPPER TRUNK EXTENSION

Muscles Stretched: Rectus abdominus (front stomach), external obliques (sides of the stomach), the pectoralis major (chest), and the serratus anterior (rib cage).

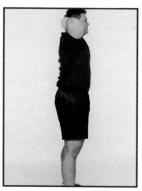 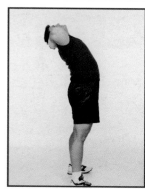

Method: From a seated or standing position, clasp hands behind head and contract erector spinae muscles. Slowly and carefully, extend trunk backward to point of maximum stretch.

Repetitions: 8-10.

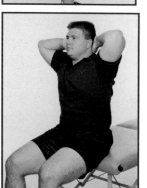 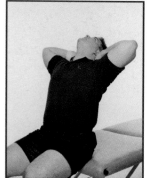

UPPER TRUNK EXTENSION: OBLIQUE

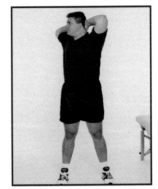
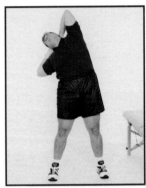
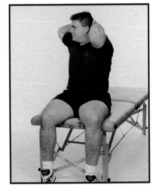
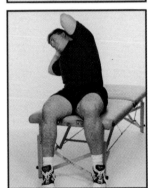

Introduction: In this variation of the previous exercise, you can isolate one side of the muscles being stretched.

Method: Rotate trunk 45 degrees and extend backward. Contract back muscles on opposite side of muscles being stretched (i.e., contract the left side back to stretch right side anterior muscles). Do not allow pelvis to rotate.

Notes: The left side obliques, serratus anterior, and intercostales will be stretched more thoroughly if you put the left side arm vertical and behind your head. Assume exact opposite position to stretch right side obliques.

Repetitions: 8-10 each side.

BENT KNEE TRUNK FLEXION

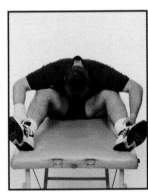

Muscles Stretched: Erector spinae and sacrospinalis muscles.

Caution: Use care if your back has been injured or surgically repaired or if you are inflexible.

Method: Begin from upright sitting position. Flex knees 4-6 inches, tuck chin, exhale, and firmly contract the abdominals as you curl your body forward. Do not bounce or make rapid movements at the end of the active stretch. At that point use your hands to assist the stretch as you continue to contract stomach muscles. Move back to starting position and repeat. Exercise may also be done sitting on a chair or in a standing position if same principles are applied.

Repetitions: 10-15.

ADVANCED TRUNK ROTATION

Muscles Stretched: Cervical, thoracic, and lumbar rotators.

Method: Sit with one leg straight. Flex the opposite knee 90 degrees and cross foot over and rest calf on the far side of straight knee. Place opposite side elbow on outside of flexed knee. Rest opposite hand behind back. Turn head and trunk as far away as possible from midline contracting opposite side cervical thoracic and lumbar rotators and assist with elbow pressure against knee. Release, face forward, repeat. Perform exercise on opposite side.

Repetitions: 8-10 each side.

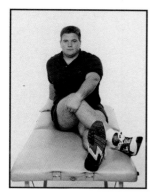 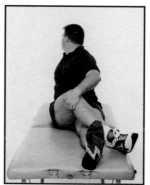 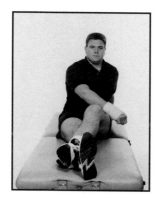 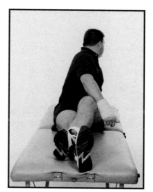

THORACIC-LUMBAR ROTATION

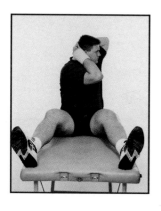 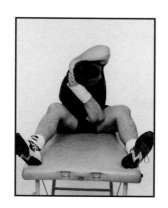 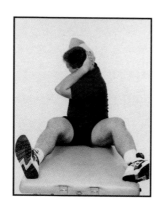 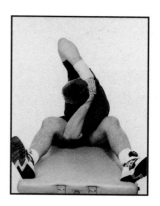

Muscles Stretched: Rotators, erector spinae and sacrospinalis — muscles and connective tissue that may limit rotation of the thoracic-lumbar spine.

Muscles Contracted: Rectus abdominus external and internal oblique muscles.
From a seated position with your feet slightly apart, clasp hands behind your head, flex knees 4-6 inches, tuck chin, and rotate trunk as far as possible in one direction. Move lower (lead) elbow around towards opposite side of trunk. Exhale and flex trunk forward, bringing lead shoulder down between the knees toward the surface. Return to starting position, complete repetitions and change sides.

Repetitions: 10 each side.

LATERAL TRUNK FLEXION (SEATED OR STANDING)

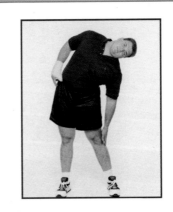
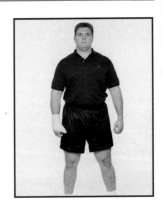

Muscles Stretched: Lateral spine flexors, quadratus lumborum (lateral), obliques, and erector spinae muscles.

Muscles Contracted: Muscles on opposite side of those to be stretched.

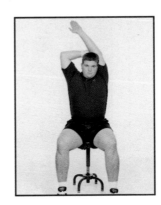
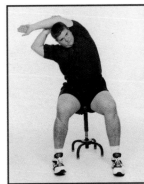

Method: Begin in a standing position with feet shoulder width, apart, knees extended, and pelvis horizontally level. Slowly bend laterally (sideways) directly over the pelvis as far as possible. Return to starting position and repeat on same side or on other side.

Notes: By placing the same side arm in a sideward elevated position (vertical), the serratus posterior and latissimus dorsi muscles receive greater stretch.

Repetitions: One or two sets of 10 repetitions for each side.

OBLIQUE LATERAL TRUNK FLEXION

Introduction: In this variation of the previous exercise, you can achieve greater isolation of the quadratus lumborum.

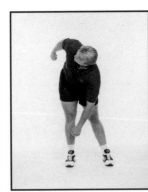

Method: Rotate the trunk 45 degrees anterior without allowing pelvis to also rotate. Contract abdominals and anterior oblique muscles diagonal to the posterior obliques being stretched. Bend at 45-degree angle obliquely in direction the front shoulder is pointed. Repeat and then stretch the other side.

Repetitions: One or two sets of 10 each side.

ANKLE-FOOT FLEXIBILITY

Stretching helps establish full range of motion for the ankle, the subtalar (a joint between the ankle bone and the heel) and metatarsal-phalangeal (the joints from the ankle to the toes) joints. It also assists in reducing problems such as calf injuries, shin splints, achilles tendon injuries, foot stress, hammer toes, and ankle and arch sprains or strains. In addition, the following flexibility exercises can increase the performance potential for sports where the lower leg muscles are involved, especially those muscles related to lateral mobility. Lower leg circulation can also be improved through some of these stretching exercises.

DORSAL ANKLE STRETCH

Muscles Stretched: Tibialis anterior and extensor digitorum muscles.

Muscles Contracted: Plantaris, soleus, gastrocnemius, and flexor digitorum muscles.

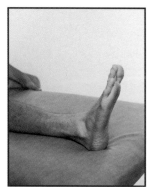 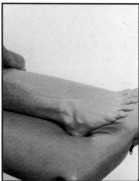

Introduction: Ankle plantar flexion (pointing the foot away from the body) may be limited because of injury, conditions causing weakness of the plantar flexors, or general lack of flexibility due to heredity, inactivity, or soreness. Over stress of these muscles may result in shin splints or tendonitis. Limited plantar flexion may be the result of a shortened tibialis anterior or tight fascia. Regular stretching of these muscles will increase plantar flexion and assist in the development of greater power and speed in sports.

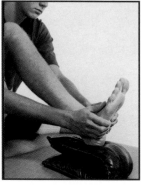 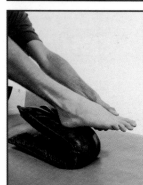

Method: Plantar flex the ankle-foot downward (toes pointing toward the surface) by contracting the plantaris, soleus, gastrocnemius, and flexor digitorum muscles and stretching the tibialis anterior and extensor digitorum muscles.

Advanced Positions: Additional stretch of the anterior tibialis will be accomplished by supinating (turning inward and downward) the foot at the end of ankle plantar flexion. You may bend the knee and assist stretch with hands. Release to beginning position and repeat.

Repetitions: One or two sets of 10.

SOLEUS STRETCH

Muscles Stretched: Soleus.

Muscles Contracted: Ankle-foot dorsal flexor muscles. Tibialis anterior, extensor digitorums.

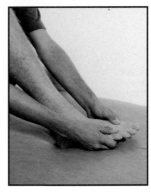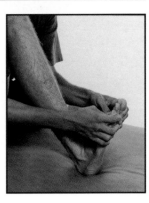

Introduction: Although a shortened soleus muscle or achilles tendon is an infrequent problem, it sometimes occurs following injury such as fracture, sprain, casting, or nerve damage.

Method: To stretch the soleus, flex knee to 90 degrees or more and lift the foot with the ankle-foot dorsal flexor muscles. Place hands under ball of foot. Provide gentle assisting stretch with the hands. Brace chest on knee for greater leverage. Release and repeat.

Notes: Flexing the knee at 90 degrees or more enables stretching without interference of the gastrocnemius muscle. This exercise is ideal as a warm-up exercise before activity or competition.

Repetitions: 8-10.

ACHILLES TENDON STRETCH

Muscles Stretched: Achilles tendon.

Muscles Contracted: Anterior tibialis and extensor digitorums.

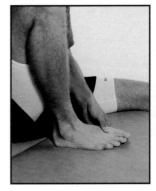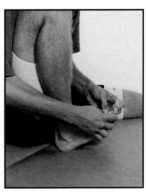

Method: For greatest isolation of achilles tendon, move foot as close to buttock as possible. From this position the ankle plantar flexors are immobilized. Dorsi flex the foot (move toes/foot toward shin) by contracting the anterior tibialis and extensor digitorums. Brace chest on knee for greater leverage. Place hands under the ball of the foot and assist at end of the active movement. Release to starting position and repeat.

Repetitions: One or two sets of 10.

GASTROCNEMIUS (CALF) STRETCH

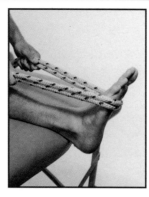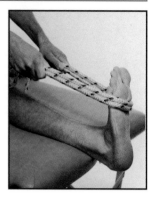

Muscles Stretched: Gastrocnemius.

Muscles Contracted: Quadriceps to lock knee joint. Anterior tibialis and extensor digitorums to lift ankle-foot.

Introduction: This heel cord stretch lengthens the two-joint gastrocnemius muscle, reducing the risk of calf pulls, shin splints, achilles tendon problems, and foot-ankle injuries.

Method: Keep knee locked by contracting quadriceps muscles. Bending the knee or leaning the upper body backwards will decrease effectiveness of this stretch. Pull foot back with anterior foot-ankle muscles, including the tibialis anterior and extensor digitorum. Assist with strap, rope, or hand. Do not pull with strap, rope, or hand unless anterior muscles are contracting. To provide greater stretch, gradually lean trunk forward more before increasing backward angle of foot-ankle.

Repetitions: 10 if for warm-ups; two to three sets of 10 alternately for tight calves.

OUTER GASTROCNEMIUS STRETCH

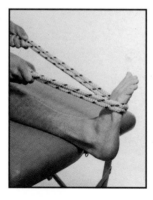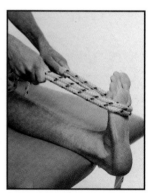

Muscles Stretched: Gastrocnemius, especially the outer belly.

Muscles Contracted: Quadriceps, anterior tibialis.

Method: To isolate the outer part of the gastrocnemius muscle, keep the knee locked, turn foot inward and lift ankle backwards. Use a rope to assist at end of the movement. Gradually lean upper body forward for greater stretch.

Repetitions: One or two sets of 10.

INNER GASTROCNEMIUS STRETCH

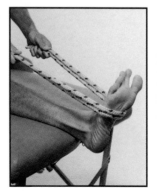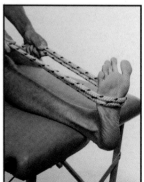

Muscles Stretched: Gastrocnemius, especially the inner part.

Muscles Contracted: Quadriceps, anterior tibialis.

Method: To stretch inner belly of gastrocnemius, keep knee locked, turn foot outward and lift ankle backwards. Use rope to assist at end of movement. Gradually lean upper body forward for greater stretch.

Repetitions: One or two sets of 10.

EVERTOR STRETCH

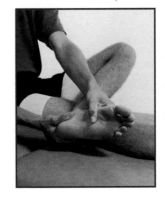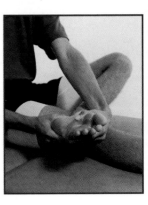

Muscles Stretched: Lateral tissue of the subtalar and foot regions including the peroneus longus, peroneus brevis, peroneus tertius, and extensor digitorum longus.

Muscles Contracted: Subtalar and foot invertor (medial) muscles, including the tibialis posterior and tibialis anterior.

Method: Begin with ankle dorsi flex to near 90 degrees and turn the ankle inward as far as possible, gradually decreasing the degree of dorsal flexion to insure greater stretching of outer forefoot pronators. Turn foot and ankle inward. Apply gentle assistance with hands positioned around heel and forefoot. Release and repeat.

Repetitions: 10.

INVERTOR STRETCH

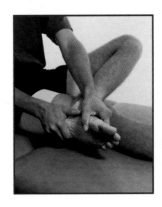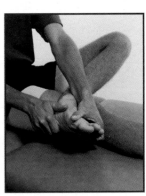

Muscles Stretched: Medial ankle muscles including the tibialis posterior and tibialis anterior.

Muscles Contracted: Lateral subtalar and foot muscles, including the peroneus longus, peroneus brevis, peroneus tertius, and extensor digitorum longus.

Method: While maintaining slight dorsal flexion of foot and ankle, turn subtalar and foot outward as far as possible by contracting lateral subtalar foot muscles. Bend knee 90 degrees, place hands around heel and forefoot, and assist at end of active effort. Gradually plantar flex (move foot away from body) ankle and pronate (turn outward and upward) the forefoot to stretch foot supinators.

Repetitions: 8-10.

FOOT PRONATOR STRETCH

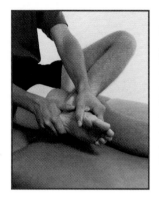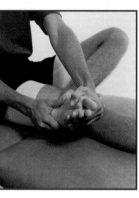

Muscles Stretched: Intrinsic dorsal muscles of the forefoot.

Muscles Contracted: Gastrocnemius, soleus and tibialis posterior.

Introduction: In skills such as jumping and rapid starting, maximum foot supination is important. The final stage of pushoff is more powerful if full range of supination is possible.

Method: Bend the knee, plantar flex ankle (flex downward), and turn foot inward as far as possible using medial lower leg musculature. Prevent sub-talar joint substitution by stabilizing heel with opposite hand. Apply gentle stretch with the hand placed around the front of foot. Release and repeat.

Repetitions: 10.

FOOT SUPINATOR STRETCH

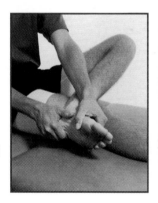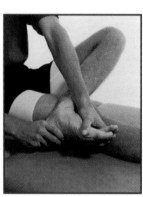

Muscles Stretched: Intrinsic plantar muscles of the forefoot.

Muscles Contracted: Peroneus longus, peroneus brevis, peroneus tertius, and extensor digitorum longus.

Introduction: People with foot problems may have limited movement of the forefoot. If the foot cannot pronate outward because of limited range, foot posture will be affected by walking on the outside of foot, perhaps resulting in pain.

Method: With the knee bent 90 degrees, dorsiflex (lift) the ankle upward, turn the foot outward as far as possible. Stabilize the heel with one hand to prevent sub-talar substitution. With the opposite hand around the forefoot, provide assisting stretch. Release and repeat.

Repetitions: 10.

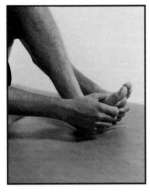
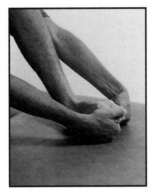

Muscles Stretched: Metatarsal arch anterior.

Muscles Contracted: Tibialis anterior to dorsi flex the ankle, flexor digitorum longus, and flexor hallucis longus to flex all toes downward.

Introduction: This stretch provides relief for the uncomfortable effects of hammered toes and tight dorsal metatarsal muscles and tendons.

Method: Dorsal flex the ankle by contracting tibialis anterior muscle. To assist in greater movement, bend knee 90 degrees, flex toes downward, and manually assist stretch with hands. Release and repeat.

Repetitions: 10-15 for warm-ups. Two or three sets of 10 for therapeutic considerations.

Additional Techniques: If an individual phalangeal joint is flexed downward, stabilize the joint with the thumb and forefinger of one hand and use the opposite hand to increase extension of the flexed joint. For overlapped toes, stabilize the toe next to the affected phalange and assist in spreading and/or rotating the toe in the opposite direction.

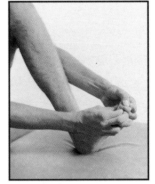
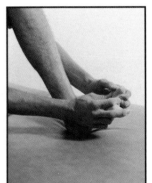

Repetitions: One or two sets of 10 frequently.

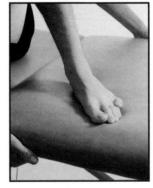
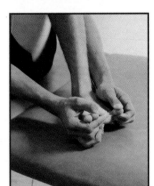

GREAT (BIG) TOE STRETCH (FLEXORS)

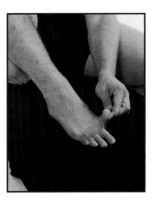

Muscles Stretched: Flexor hallucis brevis and flexor hallucis longus.

Muscles Contracted: Extensor hallucis brevis and extensor hallucis longus.

Introduction: An inability to extend the great toe affects balance, coordination, speed, ability to push off properly, and length of stride. Athletes who do extensive training and wear foot orthotics that provide firm support, but limit foot movement, will lose foot mobility unless they consistently perform foot flexibility and strength exercises.

Method: Extend big toe upward by contracting muscles on top of big toe. Assist movement gently, stretch, and release. Beware of great tissue sensitivity.

Repetitions: Two sets of 10.

GREAT (BIG) TOE STRETCH (EXTENSORS)

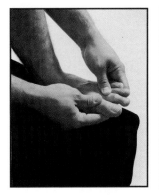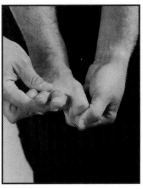

Muscles Stretched: Extensor hallucis longus and extensor hallucis brevis.

Muscles Contracted: Flexor hallucis longus and flexor hallucis brevis.

Introduction: Inflexible big toe extensors and tight achilles tendon, soleus, or gastrocnemius muscles will lead to limited foot plantar flexion. A weak anterior tibialis muscle may also cause this problem. This will affect speed, balance, ability to push off properly, length of stride, and coordination. Conditions such as hammer toe, claw foot, metatarsalgia (chronic pain in the bones connecting the ankle to the toes), and abnormally high arch may result from limited great toe flexion.

Method: Flex (bend) the big toe downward contracting the muscles on the bottom (plantar surface) of the big toe. Gently assist the movement, remembering the muscle and tendon will be quite sensitive. Assist , release, and repeat.

Repetitions: One to three sets of 10.

GREAT (BIG) TOE STRETCH (ADDUCTORS)

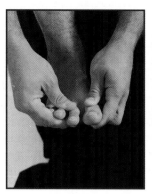 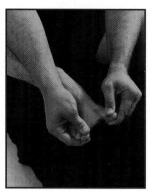 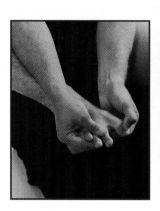

Muscles Stretched: Adductor hallucis, extensor hallucis longus, and extensor hallucis brevis.

Muscles Contracted: Abductor hallucis.

Introduction: Quite often we see a condition in which the largest toe is angled inward (hallux valgus). This condition may be uncomfortable and lead to formation of a bunion. The adductor hallucis muscle pulls the big toe towards the second toe. If the abductor hallucis is too weak to keep the toe in the normal neutral position, it will angle inward, especially if aided by the force of the shoe. Hallux valgus affects speed, balance, ability to push off properly, length of stride, and coordination. This stretch helps eliminate the inward angling of the big toe and helps prevent the major cause of a bunion. It also often positively affects a bunion that already exists by helping restore the posture of the big toe.

Method: Stabilize the four toes with one hand. Attempt to spread big toe laterally away from other toes contracting the abductor hallucis muscle. Assist the stretching of the adductor hallucis muscle at the end of active movement. To stretch the extensor hallucis longus and extensor hallucis brevis, flex the big toe downward using the flexor hallucis longus and flexor hallucis brevis. Assist movement with thumb and index finger of free hand (see previous Big Toe Extensor Stretch). For maximum stretch of big toe extensors and adductors follow by stretching extensors and adductors of big toe with a combination downward and outward stretch.

Caution: Assist gently because joint, muscles, connective tissue, scar tissue, or nerve endings will be sensitive. Joint and muscle distortion take time to correct. Release and repeat.

Repetitions: Two or three sets of 10.

LITTLE TOE STRETCH

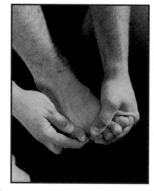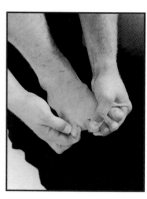

Muscles Stretched: Flexor digitorum longus.

Introduction: Frequently the little toe is postured in the shoe in a position of flexion, hyperadduction, and medial rotation. This fifth toe slides under the fourth toe rendering both functionally limited and placing greater stress on the medial foot and arches.

Method: Attempt to lift the little toe upward, contracting the extensor digitorum longus. Isolate the area, placing the thumb and index finger proximal to the affected digit. Assist the active effort with the remaining thumb and index finger. To stretch the adductor (web) portion on the toe, try to spread the toe, stabilize the adjoining toe, and assist in spreading of the little toe. If the toe is also rotating inward, mildly de-rotate toe in opposite direction.

Caution: Do these stretches slowly, as connective tissue will usually be very short.

Repetitions: Two or three sets of 10 according to the condition of the toe.

ASSISTED ACTIVE ISOLATED STRETCHING

When joints, muscles, and connective tissue lack complete range of motion, it is advantageous to have assistance in stretching. Assistance offers greater accuracy and more encouragement for the patient. Assisted stretching is especially important following neurological damage, injury, or postfracture and postoperative conditions. Some movements are difficult to perform effectively without assistance, especially when the antagonist muscles are too weak to provide enough force to move the joints or when pain is a significant factor. However, whenever possible assisted stretching should follow the patient's own active movement.

An assistant can accurately guide the movement and assist the stretching process by releasing the external pressure as the stretch reflex signals, then causing the movement to cease, and finally making sure the muscle is returned to the neutral (starting) position.

This assisted movement facilitates voluntary neural stimulation of the agonist muscles, which causes a shortening contraction of the muscles on the opposite side of the joint and tissues that are to be lengthened. The muscles and fascia are lengthened by a consistent opposite side muscle contraction that is gently assisted to the point of slight tissue discomfort, which activates the stretch reflex. Active movement insures increased circulation, oxygen and nutrition to the tissues, safety, and reciprocal cooperation between agonist and antagonist muscle groups. In addition, metabolic waste is removed from entrapped tissues as circulation increases to the area.

The assistant must be focused and concentrate so that the movement is performed safely and accurately. The assistant encourages successful stretching through constant verbal instruction and feedback and by motivating the subject to exert maximum effort. The assistant must be careful about the length of time the stretch is maintained (a maximum of 1 1/2 to 2 seconds) and amount of force provided. Preventing overstretching is accomplished by releasing the movement when signaled in order to prevent reversal contraction of the tissues being stretched (stretch reflex).

NECK FLEXIBILITY: ASSISTED

NECK STRETCHING: ASSISTED GRAVITY

Introduction: Assisted neck flexibility exercises are intended to aid people who have suffered a strain, sprain, or postfracture that has healed properly and who have obtained medical authorization to begin assisted neck flexibility and strengthening exercises.

Method: The subject moves head against gravity and is guided by the therapist in the correct plane and gently assisted where necessary. The therapist counterbalances whatever the patient cannot control without excessive muscle strain. This series of exercises also specifically strengthens the agonist muscles moving the head.

CERVICAL HYPEREXTENSION

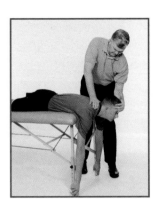

Muscles Strengthened: Upper erector spinae, splenius cervicus, splenius capitus, semispinalis cervicus and capitus.

Muscles Stretched: Sternocleidomastoid and prevertebral muscles.

Method: In the prone position with the neck extended beyond the end of the table, the subject grasps the legs of the table to keep the movement localized in the cervical spine. The therapist stands at the side of the patient, placing one hand under the forehead and the other hand on the upper thoracic spine to prevent thoracic movement. The hand on the forehead guides the head in the sagittal plane and assists stretch at the end of active movement. Exercise through full range of motion, stretch gently and repeat. Use great care with herniated disc conditions or posttraumatic neck.

Repetitions: Begin with 5 to 8 and gradually increase to 15 when subject is ready.

CERVICAL LATERAL FLEXION: RIGHT

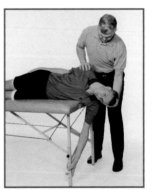 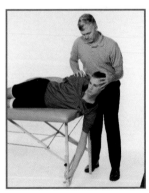

Muscles Contracted: Three scaleni, sternocleidomastoid, erector spinae, and prevertebral muscles.

Muscles Stretched: Three scaleni, sternocleidomastoid, erector spinae, and prevertebral muscles on the opposite side.

Method: Subject assumes a side-lying position with neck beyond the end of the table and lower hand grasping a table leg. Therapist stands behind patient placing hands on both sides of the head. The patient begins the exercise with the head near the left shoulder. The therapist guides the head to prevent forward movement, backward movement, or rotation. The subject moves the head (ear toward shoulder) as far as possible; a gentle assistance is then provided by the therapist. Return to starting position and repeat.

Compensation Check: To prevent shrugging of top shoulder by levator scapula muscle (compensation), therapist may place upper hand on top of the shoulder.

Repetitions: Begin with 5 to 8 and gradually increase to 15 when subject is ready.

CERVICAL ROTATION: RIGHT

Muscles Strengthened: Right sternocleidomastoid, deep posterior spinal muscles, longissimus cervicus, splenius capitus, splenius cervicus, and erector spinae muscles.

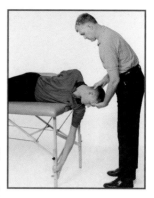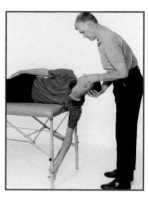

Muscles Stretched: The same muscles on the left side.

Method: Ask client to assume a side-lying position with the neck beyond the end of the table and the lower hand clasped on the table leg. Therapist stands near the top of the patient's head and places hands on the forehead and back of the head to help counterbalance the weight of the head and prevent flexion, hyperextension, or lateral flexion. Client should rotate head from downward position slowly upward (right) with therapist assisting the stretch at end of active movement

Compensation Check: To prevent top shoulder from being shrugged by levator scapula muscle you should place one hand on the shoulder.

Repetitions: Begin 5 to 8 repetitions and increase to 15 when subject is ready.

CERVICAL LATERAL FLEXION: LEFT

Muscles Stretched: Three scaleni, sternocleidomastoid, erector spinae, and prevertebral muscles.

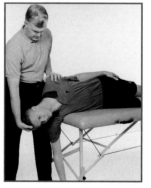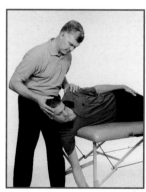

Muscles Contracted: Opposite side antagonist muscles.

Method: Subject assumes a side-lying position with neck beyond the end of the table and lower hand grasping a table leg. Therapist stands behind patient and places hands on both sides of the head. The patient begins the exercise with the head near the right shoulder. The therapist guides the head to prevent forward movement, backward movement, or rotation. The subject moves (ear to shoulder) the head as far as possible and then gentle assistance is provided by the therapist. Return to starting position and repeat.

Compensation Check: Be aware of shoulder shrug compensation, which frequently happens. You may place upper hand on top of shoulder to prevent compensation.

Repetitions: Begin with 5 to 8 and gradually increase to 15 when subject is ready.

CERVICAL ROTATION: LEFT

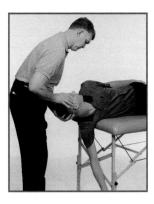

Muscles Stretched: Left sternocleidomastoid, deep posterior spinal muscles, longissimus cervicus, splenius capitus, splenius cervicus, and erector spinae muscle.

Muscles Contracted: The same muscles on the right side.

Method: From a side-lying position, subject should extend the neck beyond the end of the table and grasp a table leg with the lower hand. Therapist stands in front of the patient's head, placing the hands on the forehead and back of the head to help counterbalance the weight of the head and prevent flexion, extension, or lateral flexion. Subject rotates head from downward position slowly upward (left) with therapist guiding and assisting stretch at end of active movement.

Compensation Check: Make the patient aware of shoulder shrug compensation. You may place upper hand on top of shoulder to prevent compensation.

Repetitions: Begin 5 to 8 repetitions and increase to 15 when subject is ready.

CERVICAL FLEXION: SUPINE

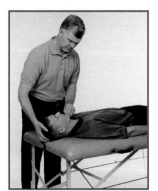
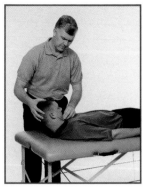

Muscles Stretched: Upper erector spinae, splenius cervicus, splenius capitus, semispinalis cervicus and semispinalis capitus.

Muscles Contracted: Sternocleidomastoid and prevertebral muscles.

Method: Ask subject to assume a supine position with head on table. Shoulders and upper back should remain on the table throughout this exercise. Therapist stands at side of patient with one hand behind the upper-posterior head and the other hand around lower border of jaw. From the neutral position, ask subject to tuck the chin as close as possible near the neck and lift head in a close tuck without allowing the thoracic spine to leave surface. Therapist assists subject in tucking chin, counterbalances weight of head, if needed, and provides gentle assistance at end of active movement. Slowly return to starting position and repeat.

Repetitions: Begin 5 to 8 repetitions and gradually increase to 15 when subject is ready.

NECK FLEXIBILITY ASSISTED: STANDING

Frequently, the cervical spine (neck) has decreased range of motion due to age, postinjury, surgery, muscle tension, or postural deficiencies. Exercise caution with disc problems, calcium deposits, or osteoporosis.

ANTERIOR SEMI-CIRCLES

Introduction: This motion provides a gentle warm up and increases blood flow prior to the following specific movements. To prevent aggravation of cervical ligaments or endanger blood vessels or nerves, do not complete full circle going in back of neutral position.

Method: Begin by moving chin toward one shoulder, then lower chin as you move toward breast bone (sternum), continue in upward movement toward opposite shoulder. Repeat moving chin toward sternum and up toward opposite shoulder. This movement is similar to a pendulum on a grandfather's clock. Therapist may need to guide movement.

Repetitions: 8 to 10.

CERVICAL FLEXION

Muscles Stretched: Cervical (neck) extensor muscles, including the multifidus, semispinalis, oblique capitus, and erector spinae.

Muscles Contracted: Anterior neck muscles (flexors), including the rectus capitus anterior, rectus capitus lateralis, sternocleidomastoid, longus colli, longus capitus, and scalene muscles.

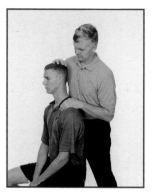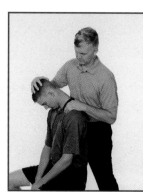

Method: Instruct the subject to tuck the chin as close to the neck as possible and contract the anterior neck muscles (flexors). Therapist assists the end of the movement. Release to starting position and repeat.

Repetitions: 10 to 15.

CERVICAL EXTENSION

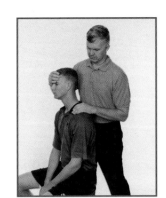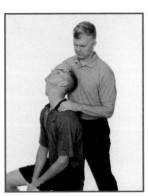

Muscles Stretched: Cervical flexor muscles including the longus colli, longus capitus, rectus capitus anterior, rectus capitus lateralis, and scalene muscles.

Muscles Contracted: Multifidus, semispinalis, oblique capitus and erector spinae.

Method: Instruct the subject to contract the posterior neck muscles (extensors) by gently tilting the head backward. Therapists assists by placing one hand at the cervical thoracic juncture and the opposite hand on subject's forehead to guide and assist. Release, return to starting position, and repeat.

Caution: Cervical extension from the vertical position may be contraindicated for pinched nerve or herniated disc. Medical approval is suggested.

Repetitions: 10.

CERVICAL LATERAL FLEXION

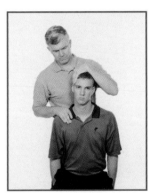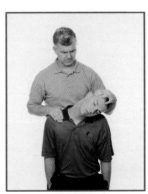
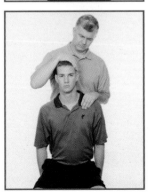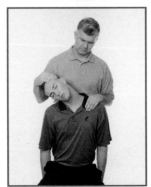

Muscles Stretched: Side lateral flexors — three scalene, sternocleidomastoid, and splenius capitus muscles.

Muscles Contracted: Opposite side scalene muscles, sternocleidomastoid, and splenius capitus.

Method: This exercise may be performed in the sitting or supine postures. Ask subject to contract the muscles on the opposite side of those being stretched. Give gentle assistance for two seconds with free hand at end of movement. Release to starting position and repeat.

Compensation Check: Therapist should stabilize the shoulder on the side being stretched to prevent compensation of a lower spinal area or hiking of shoulder by levator scapula muscle.

Repetitions: One or two sets of 10 both sides, according to need of subject.

CERVICAL ROTATION

Muscles Stretched: Neck rotators, including the multifidus, rotators, semispinalis, and sternocleidomastoid muscles.

Muscles Contracted: Opposite side neck rotators.

Method: The exercise may be performed in a sitting or supine position. As subject rotates head in one direction as far as possible, assist movement gently with one hand on each side of the head. Have subject return to the neutral position and repeat movement.

Compensation Check: Keep head in neutral position and attempt to prevent neck compensation by lateral flexion or hyperextension. To prevent rotation of the shoulder girdle complex, keep left shoulder back when rotating right and right shoulder stable when rotating left.

Repetitions: One or two sets of 10, both directions.

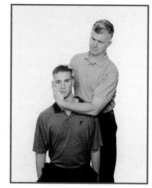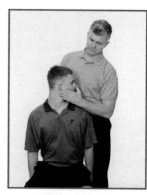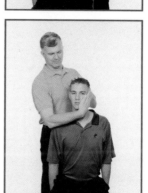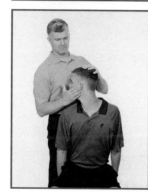

CERVICAL ANTERIOR OBLIQUE

Muscles Stretched: Upper trapezius, which moves the neck and head posterior and lateral. The semispinalis capitus, longissimus capitus, erector spinae, and middle and posterior scalenes are also isolated.

Muscles Contracted: Rectus capitus anterior, rectus capitus lateralis, sternocleidomastoid, longus colli, longus capitus, and middle and anterior scalene muscles.

Introduction: Tight trapezius and levator scapula muscles are a major source of cervical tension. This exercise may be performed from the sitting or supine positions.

Method: In order to stretch the left side, the subject will rotate the head 45 degrees to the left, then move the head to the right antero-laterally (obliquely) at a 45 degree angle (right ear toward right breast). Guide the movement and gently assist the stretch. Release, move back to neutral position, and repeat. To stretch the right side, rotate the head 45 degrees to the right. The head is moved to the left anterolateral, obliquely at a 45 degree angle (left ear toward left breast). Guide the movement and assist with a gentle assist from therapist. Release to neutral position and repeat.

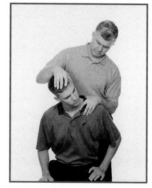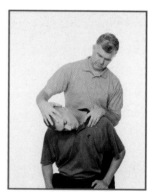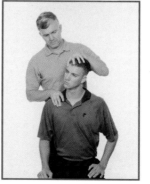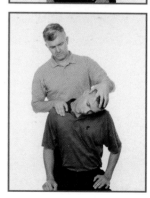

Repetitions: One or two sets of 10.

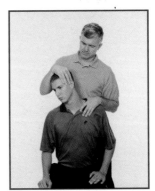
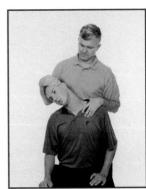

Muscles Stretched: Right anterior scalenus, sternocleidomastoid, longus colli cervicis, longus capitus, and rectus capitus.

Muscles Contracted: Left cervical extensors including the multifidus, semispinalis, oblique capitus, and erector spinae.

Notes: This exercise may be performed from a seated, supine, or prone position.

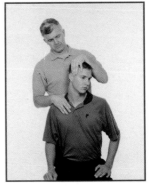
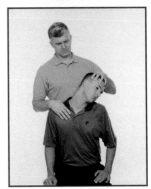

Method: Subject should rotate the head to the left 45 degrees moving postero-obliquely at a 45 degree angle, ear toward outer border of shoulder blade. At the end of active movement, the therapist gently assists the movement for two seconds. Release to the neutral position and repeat. The left side flexors are isolated by rotating the head to the right 45 degrees and moving the head postero-obliquely toward the outside of the right scapula.

Compensation Check: Therapist may stabilize shoulder on side of muscles being stretched.

Repetitions: One or two sets of 10.

SHOULDER FLEXIBILITY: ASSISTED

Assisted shoulder flexibility exercises stretch the glenohumeral, acromioclavicular, sternoclavicular joints, the scapular musculature, and the connective tissue. Greater flexibility will help prevent injuries, aid postinjury or postsurgical recovery, and enhance performance of the shoulder region. For more details concerning the following exercises, which show where and how assistance may by beneficial, consult the Shoulder Flexibility: Active section of this book.

SHOULDER CIRCUMDUCTION

Introduction: Circumduction increases circulation in the shoulder complex and arm.

Method: Initiate arm circles toward and away from body midline. Arms should hang like wet noodles when performing bent-over circumduction. Lean body forward, bend knees, and tighten stomach muscles. Begin with small circles and increase in circumference. Patient may do giant (circumduction) arm circles from standing position if shoulder is not sore or injured.

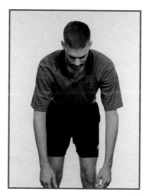 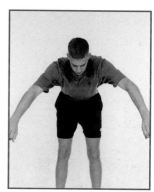

Repetitions: 10 to 15 repetitions in each direction.

HORIZONTAL EXTENSION I

Muscles Stretched: Pectoralis major and pectoralis minor

Muscles Contracted: Rhomboids major and minor and trapezius II, III, and IV.

Introduction: This exercise is important for full horizontal shoulder range of motion and improves throwing and over-head striking movements.

Method: Ask subject to begin with palms together and elbows extended in front of chest. Instruct subject to reach back as far as possible and then offer gentle assistance. Release and repeat. As muscles loosen, ask subject to raise arms higher to stretch upper pectoral fibers.

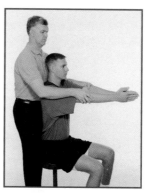 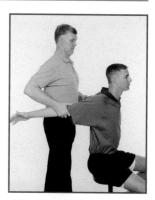

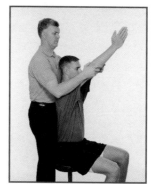 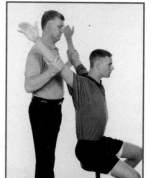

Repetitions: 10 to 15.

HORIZONTAL EXTENSION II

Muscles Stretched: Same as previous exercise but stretches upper pectoral (clavicular) fibers more completely.

Muscles Contracted: Rhomboid and trapezius muscles.

Method: Ask subject to interlock fingers behind the head. Assist gently at end of movement as the subject reaches elbows backward, contracting rhomboid and trapezius muscles.

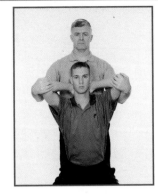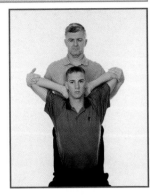

Repetitions: 8 to 10.

SHOULDER HYPEREXTENSION: SINGLE ARMS

Muscles Stretched: Long head of biceps brachii, anterior deltoids, and pectoralis major and minor.

Muscles Contracted: Triceps and posterior deltoids.

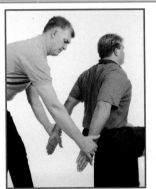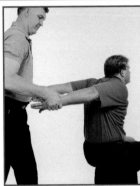

Introduction: This stretch is especially beneficial for post-surgery, postinjury, or extreme tightness. Patient should stand or sit without bending body forward. Instruct subject to extend arms backward with elbows locked. Ask subject to reach back as far as possible, contracting triceps and posterior deltoids. Provide gentle assistance, release, and repeat.

Repetitions: 10.

SHOULDER HYPEREXTENSION: HANDS CLASPED

Muscles Stretched: Short head of biceps brachii, pectoralis major and minor, and anterior deltoids.

Muscles Contracted: Triceps and posterior deltoids.

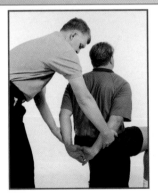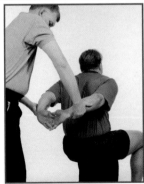

Method: From a standing or sitting position, without bending body forward, ask subject to reach arms upward as far a possible, lock elbows, and interlace fingers with palms of hands facing away from body. Subject should reach back as far as possible contracting triceps and posterior deltoids. Provide gentle assistance, release, and repeat.

Compensation Check: For the most effective stretching, attempt to keep scapulae from moving toward spine during the movement. If necessary, this may be accomplished by having the assistant keep one hand placed between the subject's shoulder blades.

Repetitions: One or two sets of 10.

HORIZONTAL EXTENSION: POSTERIOR

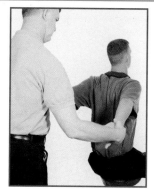
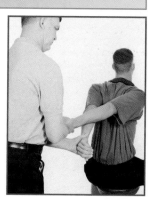

Muscles Stretched: Pectoral proximal (humerus) attachment and anterior deltoid.

Muscles Contracted: Rhomboid major, rhomboid minor, and trapezius.

Notes: Do this stretch following the Shoulder Hyperextension: Single Arm.

Method: Instruct patient to horizontally adduct scapulae contracting rhomboid major, rhomboid minor, and trapezius muscles. With subject's palms facing each other, have subject move hands horizontally backward toward posterior midline. Assist movement with brief stretch, release, and repeat until shortened fibers are free.

Repetitions: Minimum 8-10.

SHOULDER: EXTERNAL ROTATION

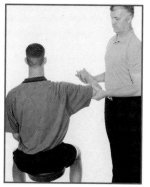
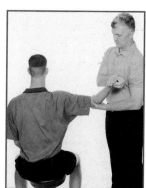

Muscles Stretched: Internal shoulder rotators, including the pectoralis major, subscapularis, latissimus dorsi and teres major.

Muscles Contracted: Superspinatis, infraspinatis, and teres minor (posterior rotator cuff).

Method: Instruct patient to bend elbow at a 90 to 95 degree angle at shoulder height if possible. The subject should externally rotate shoulder using the infraspinatus and teres minor muscles. At end of movement, therapist should provide gentle assistance, release to starting position, and repeat.

Compensation Check: Do not allow subject to arch back or rotate upper body in opposite direction.

Repetitions: 10.

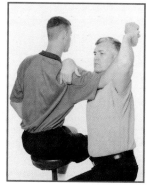
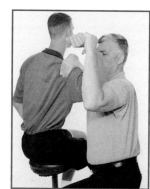

Advanced Method: To prevent compensation and provide greater isolation of the medial shoulder rotators, place hand around the posterior head of the subject's humerus (under axilla). Pull upward and then clamp wrist-forearm over anterior head of humerus. This will prevent forward compensation of humeral head. Rest subject's elbow on your chest, clasp wrist of subject. Maintain the subject's elbow at about a 95 degree angle to prevent biceps interference. Gently assist subject's active movement. Release and repeat.

Repetitions: 10-15.

SHOULDER EXTERNAL ROTATION: PRONE

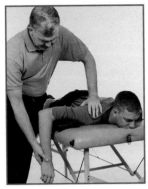 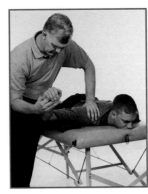

Muscles Stretched: Teres major, subscapularis, and pectoralis major muscles.

Muscles Contracted: Supraspinatus, infraspinatus, and teres minor muscles (posterior rotator cuff).

Introduction: This stretch is helpful in treating frozen or post-operative shoulders lacking external rotation.

Method: Subject assumes a prone position with the elbow bent 90 degrees and parallel to shoulder. If necessary, place a pad under the elbow so that arm is level with shoulder. Fold a towel a number of times and place it under the anterior head of humerus (front of shoulder) to prevent anterior (forward) compensation of humerus. Therapist should place stabilizing pressure on posterior head of humerus with proximal hand. Next place distal hand on wrist of patient and rest forearm on top of patient's arm to prevent patient from lifting arm during rotation. Instruct patient to reach hand upward as far as possible, then assist at end of active movement. Release to starting position and repeat.

Repetitions: One or two sets of 10.

SHOULDER EXTERNAL ROTATION: SUPINE

Muscles Stretched: Teres major, subscapularis, and pectoralis major muscles.

Muscles Contracted: Supraspinatus, infraspinatus, and teres minor muscles (posterior rotator cuff).

Introduction: For treatment of painful, frozen or post-operative shoulders with limited external rotation.

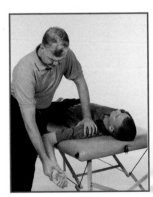

Method: Subject assumes a supine position with elbow bent 90 degrees and parallel to shoulder. With proximal hand, therapist should place stabilizing pressure on the anterior — inferior portion of head of the patient's humerus. Place distal hand on wrist of patient, and instruct subject to reach lower arm back as far as possible. Gently assist at end of active movement. Release to starting position and repeat.

Caution: Great care must be taken in this position so that the shoulder is not overstretched or dislocated.

Repetitions: One or two sets of 10.

SHOULDER: INTERNAL ROTATION

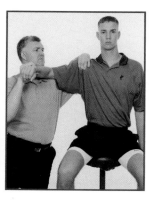 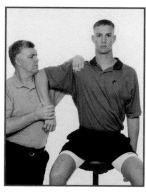

Muscles Stretched: External shoulder rotators (posterior rotator cuff) including the supraspinatus, infraspinatus and teres minor muscles.

Muscles Contracted: Internal shoulder rotators including the teres major, subscapularis, pectoralis major, and latissimus dorsi.

Method: Assistant should be in a position to stabilize scapula by placing top hand over shoulder and clasp at subject's axilla. Rest subject's elbow on your chest and stabilize the posterior head of the patient's humerus with your forearm. Assist active stretch with opposite hand. Release to starting position and repeat.

Notes: Also do Horizontal Flexion I and Horizontal Flexion II to insure maximum stretching of all posterior rotator cuff fibers.

Repetitions: One or two sets of 10, depending on patient's muscle flexibility.

SHOULDER INTERNAL ROTATION: PRONE

Muscles Stretched: Supraspinatus, infraspinatus, and teres minor (posterior rotator cuff).

Muscles Contracted: Teres major, subscapularis, and pectoralis major, and latissimus dorsi.

Introduction: This is a good technique for frozen, postinjury, or postoperative shoulders where internal rotation is limited.

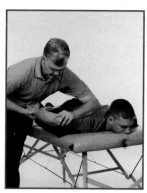

Method: Ask subject to assume a prone position. Fold small towel a number of times and place it under the front of the shoulder to prevent anterior movement of humeral head. Place patient's elbow in a position parallel to shoulder and bent 90 degrees. Place pad under the elbow to keep arm level with shoulder if necessary. Instruct subject to reach arm upward, rotating shoulder inward. To prevent compensation, stabilize the posterior head of humerus with hand and lower border of scapula with elbow. At end of active movement, assist gently with opposite hand on patient's wrist. Assist stretch, release to starting position, and repeat.

Repetitions: One or two sets of 10.

SHOULDER INTERNAL ROTATION: SUPINE

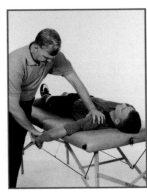

Muscles Stretched: Supraspinatus, infraspinatus, and teres minor muscles (posterior rotator cuff).

Muscles Contracted: Teres major, subscapularis, pectoralis major, and latissimus dorsi.

Method: Subject assumes a supine position with elbow bent 90 degrees and parallel to shoulder. Stabilize the anterior-superior portion of head of humerus by using pressure from your proximal hand. Place distal hand on wrist of patient. Instruct subject to rotate arm downward as far as possible, then assist at end of active movement. Release to starting position and repeat.

Caution: Great care must be taken in this position so that the shoulder is not overstretched.

Repetitions: 10.

HORIZONTAL FLEXION I

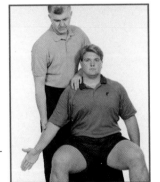 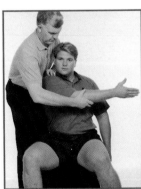

Muscles Stretched: Trapezius, rhomboid major, rhomboid minor, and the external shoulder rotators especially the infraspinatus and teres minor muscles.

Muscles Contracted: Pectoralis major, anterior deltoid, and coracobrachialis muscles.

Method: Patient should extend elbow and maintain shoulder in a parallel position, reaching arm toward opposite shoulder. Position yourself slightly behind patient and use your same side hand on the patient's elbow to assist with stretch at end of movement. Assistant may need to assist the arm movement and hold shoulder down with the other hand. Return the arm to side after each repetition.

Notes: Exercising arm must clear the top of the same side pectoral tissue.

Compensation Check: Assistant should help prevent shoulder from shrugging or moving forward from the neutral position.

Repetitions: 8 to 10.

HORIZONTAL FLEXION II

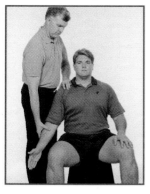 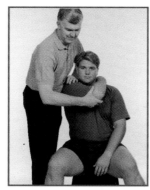

Muscles Stretched: Levator scapula and supraspinatus muscles plus the infraspinatus, teres minor, and trapezius muscles.

Muscles Contracted: Pectoralis major, teres major, subscapularis, anterior deltoid, and coracobrachialis.

Method: Instruct subject to reach around toward opposite shoulder and walk the fingers down upper back as far as possible. From a position slightly behind subject, place your same side hand on the elbow of the patient's exercising arm. Give gentle assistance at end of movement.

Compensation Check: Place your opposite side had on the exercising shoulder to prevent it from shrugging or moving forward from the neutral position. Return the arm to the patient's side after each repetition.

Repetitions: 8 to 10.

TRICEPS STRETCH: ASSISTED

Muscles Stretched: Triceps brachii, a two-joint muscle of the posterior shoulder and elbow joints.

Muscles Contracted: Biceps brachii and anterior deltoid muscles.

Introduction: It is very difficult to reach the arm completely overhead (forward elevation) unless the triceps are flexible.

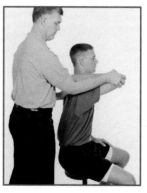 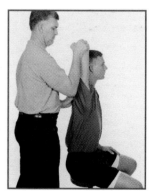

Method: Instruct the patient to flex elbow at a 90 degree position with palm facing midline. Stand behind and slightly to the side of patient and ask patient to move elbow upward. Subject should extend arm upward as far as possible with assistance. Return to starting position after each repetition.

Repetitions: 8 to 10.

SHOULDER: FORWARD ELEVATION

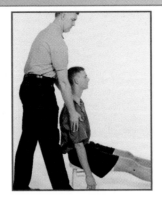
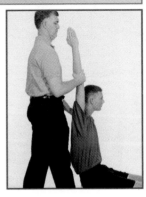

Muscles Stretched: Triceps, posterior deltoid and anterior serratus.

Muscles Contracted: Anterior deltoid and biceps brachii.

Notes: Stretch triceps and internal shoulder rotators prior to forward elevation of shoulder to allow maximal potential. Patient must be capable of a 90-degree plus external rotation in order to achieve maximal forward elevation.

Method: Ask subject to lock elbow with palm facing body. Stand behind and slightly to the side and assist with same side hand on subject's elbow. Subject raises arm as high as possible without bending elbow or arching back. Assist, release, and return to side after each repetition.

Compensation Check: To prevent shoulder from shrugging, stabilize shoulder with opposite side hand.

Advanced Stretch: In addition, athletes who require full forward elevation, should also do this stretch with the palm facing forward, and with palm facing away from body.

Repetitions: 10-15.

SHOULDER FORWARD ELEVATION: PRONE

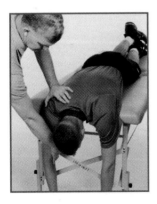
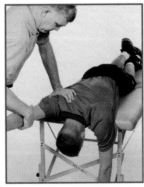

Muscles Stretched: Upper triceps, posterior deltoid, and anterior serratus.

Muscles Contracted: Anterior deltoid and biceps brachii.

Introduction: This stretch lengthens and restores full forward joint movement and is especially helpful for those with limited overhead arm movement.

Method: Ask subject to assume prone position with arms hanging off table. The shoulder should be flexed, the elbow locked, and the palm facing the body. Subject should then reach forward, contracting the anterior deltoid and biceps brachii. Assistant guides with one hand above posterior elbow joint while stabilizing the back of shoulder with the other. Return to starting position and repeat.

Repetitions: 10 to 15.

SHOULDER: SIDEWARD ELEVATION

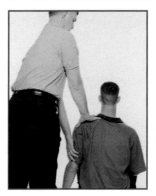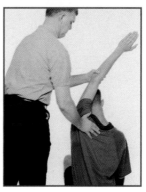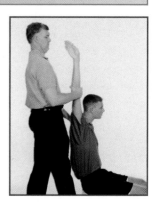

Muscles Stretched: Teres major, lattisimus dorsi, and sternal portion of the pectoralis major.

Muscles Contracted: Deltoid muscle, serratus anterior, and trapezius.

Notes: Subject must have near complete forward elevation to do this exercise.

Method: Ask subject to lock elbow, face palm forward, and reach as high as possible. Stabilize shoulder and provide assistance to movement by placing other hand above the back of the elbow. Release, return arm to the side of body, and repeat.

Compensation Check: For maximal result, do not allow elbow to bend.

Advanced Stretch: Instruct patient to externally rotate shoulder as far as comfortable and without bending elbow, reach behind head toward opposite shoulder.

Repetitions: 10.

POSTERIOR HAND CLASP

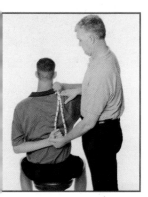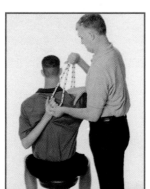

Muscles Stretched: Top arm —triceps, serratus anterior and upper pectoral fibers and the long head of biceps brachii. Lower arm — supraspinatus, infraspinatus, and teres minor.

Introduction: The goal of this stretch, the posterier clasping of hands, is often achieved slowly, and it is the therapist's job to gently assist in that goal.

Method: Position the upper arm vertically near the neck, palm facing body. As top arm reaches over (abduction) and downward (lateral rotation) the triceps, serratus anterior and upper pectoral fibers are stretched. Position the opposite hand (lower) with palm facing away from body. This hand will move up spine between shoulder blades attempting to join top hand. As lower arm reaches under (medial rotation) and upward (adduction) the long head of biceps brachii, supraspinatus, infraspinatus and teres minor are lengthened. Use rope or towel for assistance. Instruct the patient to walk the hands toward each other. At end of movement, assist the active effort by moving the lower arm upward or top arm downward.

Caution: Do not assist either movement unless active effort is sustained.

Notes: It is not unusual that a person can do this well on one side, but not the other. Work equally on the left and right side or you may experience greater risk of injuries when stressed in extended positions.

Repetitions: 8 to 10.

HIP JOINT FLEXIBILITY: ASSISTED

Increased hip flexibility helps prevent injuries and improve performance. The hip joint muscles are often limited in total range and muscle strains are frequent. Performance is limited by lack of flexibility, which affects speed and agility. Muscles of the hip are also related to problems involving the knees and lower back. Assisted stretching can improve poor hip flexibility, helps in full recovery from injuries, and increases performance in sports activities.

HAMSTRING STRETCH: BENT KNEE

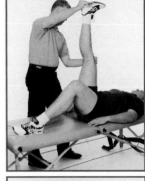

Muscles Stretched: Lower posterior thigh, distal hamstrings, semitendinosus, semimembranosus, and biceps femoris area.

Muscles Contracted: Quadriceps, including vastus medialis, vastus lateralis. vastus intermedius, and rector femoris.

Introduction: This is an effective stretch for those who are weak or have suffered from a stroke or who have muscle disease. It is also important for back, hip or hamstring histories; injury prevention; or early stages of performance improvement.

Notes: Flexion of opposite side knee is important to prevent back or hip irritation. Patients with back histories should be instructed to contract abdominals when nearing the stretch position.

Method: Ask subject to contract the anterior thigh muscles (quadriceps) and extend the knee as far as possible. Use gentle assistance. The subject may also use a rope to assist. Help patient place same side hand on knee; opposite hand will hold rope. As tissue elasticity improves, move thigh closer to the chest. For maximum stretch of lower hamstring attachments, the knee must extend completely. Release to starting position and repeat.

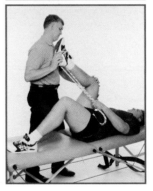
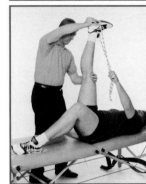

Repetitions: Two or three sets of 10 repetitions. Alternate legs after each set.

BICEPS FEMORIS STRETCH: DISTAL

Muscles Stretched: Lower biceps femoris (hamstrings).

Muscles Contracted: Quadriceps.

Method: To isolate the distal attachment of the biceps femoris, ask patient to rotate the lower leg (tibia) inward and maintain this position while extending the knee completely. Help patient place rope under foot and wrap both strands around inside of lower leg to maintain lower leg position at end of movement and assist with stretch. Release to starting position and repeat.

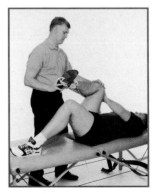
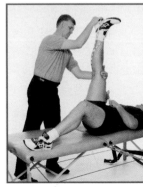

Compensation Check: Do not allow femur (thigh) to rotate inward.

Repetitions: One or two sets of 10.

SEMITENDINOSUS-SEMIMEMBRANOSUS STRETCH: DISTAL

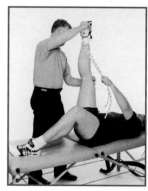

Muscles Stretched: Semitendinosus and semimembranosus (hamstrings).

Muscles Contracted: Quadriceps.

Method: To isolate the semitendinosus and semimembranosus distal attachments, rotate the lower leg (tibia) outward. Instruct subject to extend the knee completely by contracting the quadriceps. Help patient place rope under foot and both strands around outside of lower leg to maintain lower leg position and assist quadriceps muscles. Release to starting position and repeat.

Compensation Check: Do not allow the upper leg (femur) to rotate outward.

Repetitions: One or two sets of 10.

HAMSTRING STRETCH: STRAIGHT LEG

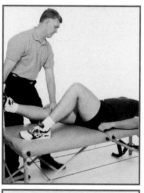
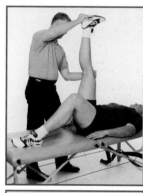
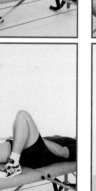
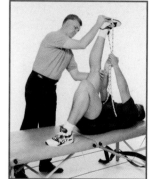

Muscles Stretched: Proximal hamstring muscles.

Muscles Contracted: Quadriceps muscles.

Introduction: This stretch provides increased upper posterior thigh and hamstring flexibility, and is an effective stretch for those who are weak or have suffered from a stroke or who have muscle disease.

Notes: This exercise may be more difficult for acute or severe back problems, but it is an important stretch for people with back, hip, or hamstring histories; for injury prevention; and for improvement of athletic performance. If back problems are present, be sure patient maintains flexion of the opposite side knee to prevent further injury or irritation.

Method: Ask patient to assume a supine position and flex the nonexercising knee. Instruct patient to lift leg by contracting the anterior thigh muscles (quadriceps). Help subject maintain a locked knee by placing your near side hand just above patella. Assist at end of active movement with other hand placed in back of lower leg (but not behind knee). If a rope is used to assist the movement, instruct subject in method of walking hands up rope.

Compensation Check: It may be necessary to place a pad and strap above the pelvis to prevent pelvic compensation. Also be aware of patient's compensation through external rotation of the femur while he/she executes lifting movement. Release and return to starting position.

Repetitions: Two or three sets of 10. Alternate legs after each set.

SEMITENDINOSUS-SEMIMEMBRANOSUS STRETCH: PROXIMAL

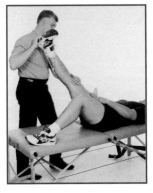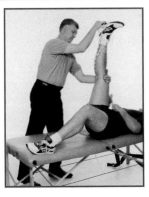

Muscles Stretched: Semitendinosus and semimembranosus (hamstrings).

Muscles Contracted: Quadriceps.

Method: To isolate the semitendinosus and semimembranosus proximal attachments, ask patient to keep knee fully extended and rotate femur (upper leg) inward. A rope may be used to assist movement. Place the rope around the bottom of foot and wrap both strands around inside of lower leg. Instruct subject to move leg toward same side shoulder by contracting quadriceps. Show subject how to assist by walking hands up the rope at end of movement, where quadriceps have least strength.

Compensation Check: Knee must not bend to get stretch of proximal end of hamstrings.

Repetitions: Two sets of 10.

BICEPS FEMORIS STRETCH: PROXIMAL

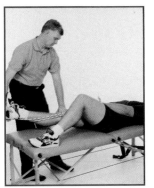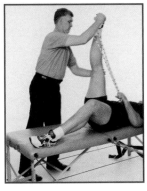

Muscles Stretched: Biceps femoris (hamstrings)

Muscles Contracted: Quadriceps

Method: To isolate the biceps femoris proximal attachment, ask patient to move noninvolved leg across midline and rotate inward and to turn exercising leg outward. Instruct subject to keep knee extended by contracting quadriceps and to contract inner thigh (hip adductor muscles) and reach toward opposite side shoulder while you provide assistance. If using rope to assist stretch, instruct patient in correct placement of rope under bottom of foot, with both strands around outside of lower leg. Show patient how to walk hands up the rope while he/she reaches with leg.

Notes: From this position, tensing the quadriceps keeps the knee straight and the hip adductors perform the movement.

Repetitions: Two sets of 10.

LATERAL HIP-THIGH STRETCH

Muscles Stretched: Lateral hip muscles including the gluteus medius, vastus lateralis, tensor fascia latae, and the iliotibial band.

Muscles Contracted: Adductors — pectineus, gracilis, adductor magnus, adductor longus, and adductor brevis.

Introduction: The muscles of the lateral hip and thigh may be tight and cause problems related to the back, hip, or knee.

Continued On Following Page

LATERAL HIP-THIGH STRETCH (CON'T.)

Method: While maintaining an extended knee, subject should externally rotate femur, and contract inner thigh muscles (adductors). Assistant helps maintain thigh angle as subject rotates nonexercising leg inward and moves across midline (hyperadduction) as far as possible. Subject may use rope to help maintain moving leg position and assist movement. Instruct patient in proper use of rope by placing it under the foot and wrapping both strands around the outside of lower leg. Then show him/her how to walk hands up the rope to assist adductor muscles.

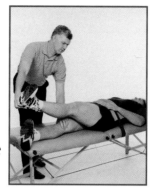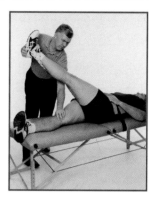

Compensation Check: A pad and seatbelt may be used to stabilize the pelvis and prevent pelvic compensation for subjects with limited hip hyperadduction movement. Return to starting position and repeat.

Repetitions: Two sets of 10.

HIP ADDUCTOR (GROIN) STRETCH: SINGLE

Muscles Stretched: Adductors — pectineus, gracilis, adductors magnus, adductor longus, and adductor brevis.

Muscles Contracted: Gluteus medius, gluteus minimus, tensor fascia latae, and sartorius.

Introduction: For situations involving extreme tightness of the groin or following a fracture or injury to the hip, stretch the adductor muscles cautiously, one leg at a time.

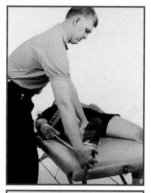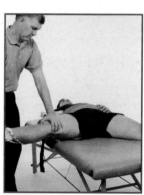

Method: Ask subject to lock knee and rotate entire leg slightly inward, spreading the leg outward as far as possible, with gentle guidance and assistance provided by the therapist. You may also wish to instruct patient in proper use of assisting with a rope by placing rope under foot and wrapping strands around inside of ankle. Return the leg to the midline and repeat.

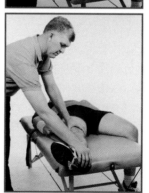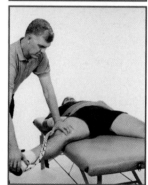

Additional Stretch: To isolate the adductor magnus most effectively, extend the knee and rotate hip 45 degrees externally, then abduct (spread) the hip and extend downward as far as possible with assistance of therapist. If using rope omit wrapping strands around inside of ankle. Return to the midline and repeat.

Compensation Check: You may prevent opposite leg from sliding by strapping leg above knee with a seatbelt or draping it over side of table.

Repetitions: One or two sets of 10, both legs.

PSOAS STRETCH

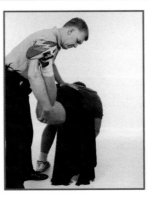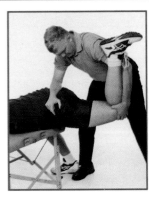

Muscles Stretched: Psoas and iliacus muscles.

Muscles Contracted: Hip extensors (gluteus maximus and proximal hamstrings).

Method: From the prone position have subject lean across table. With upper body and pelvis supported on table, place nonexercising leg about 18 inches beyond the proximal end of the table to prevent compensation by hyperextension of the back. Have subject release pressure on nonexercising leg. Maintain exercising leg at 95 to 100 degrees and keep adducted toward resting leg. Assist in keeping the resting leg in the proper position to prevent lumbar hyperextension. Place near side hand across top of pelvis to help stabilize it. Use your opposite hand to guide patient's leg through the stretching motion, helping maintain the 90 plus degree angle and the adducted position. This is accomplished by standing at the inside position and placing outside hand around lateral side of knee to prevent abduction and external rotation of exercising hip. Instruct subject to contract the gluteus maximus and hamstrings throughout movement. Assist stretch at end of range, release to starting position, and repeat.

Caution: Be sure patient does not to push on the resting leg for assistance because it may result in referred lower back discomfort.

Repetitions: One or two sets of 10 repetitions depending on amount of release.

QUADRICEPS RECTUS FEMORIS STRETCH: SIDE-LYING

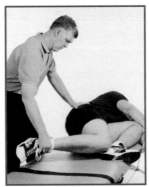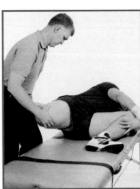

Muscles Stretched: Rectus femoris (quadriceps).

Muscles Contracted: Gluteus maximus and hamstrings.

Method: Subject assumes side-lying position and moves lower knee against chest and maintains this position by placing hand under the foot or cradling lower thigh around knee. The top hip should remain centered over the lower hip; do not allow top hip to tip backward. Exercising leg is in an adducted (thigh together) position throughout movement. If rectus femoris is very tight, subject may release pressure by using a rope to extend angle between ankle and buttocks. Assist patient in stretching the rectus femoris with three distinct stretches:

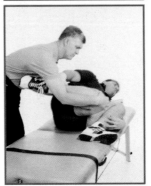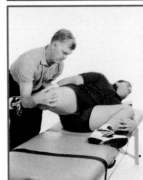

1) With top leg at 90 degree angle, place one hand in back of top hip and the other hand around subject's ankle. Instruct subject to extend thigh backward and assist.

Repetitions: Repeat 8-10.

Continued On Following Page

2) To release tension on proximal end of rectus femoris (hip flexor portion), have subject positioned with thigh in straight line with upper body. Help maintain this angle as the subject actively flexes the knee by contracting the hamstrings and moving the lower leg toward the buttocks. Assist at end of movement. Release as stretch reflex is triggered. Return to starting position (90 degree angle at knee) and repeat movement.

Repetitions: One or two sets of 10.

3) Standing behind the subject, place proximal hand across back of top hip and opposite hand in front of top thigh. Ask subject to clasp his/her top ankle and move the thigh backward with hamstrings and gluteus maximus. Instruct subject to contract abdominal muscles to prevent back hyperextension. Lower leg must also remain near chest as movement is performed. Instruct patient how to use his/her hand for an additional stretch. Release and repeat. Alternate legs after each set.

Repetitions: Two sets of 10.

RECTUS FEMORIS: PRONE

Muscles Stretched: Rectus femoris (quadriceps).

Muscles Contracted: Gluteus maximus and hamstrings.

Introduction: Serving both the knee and hip joints, the rectus femoris often becomes a shortened muscle.

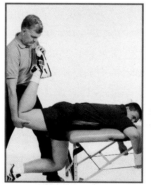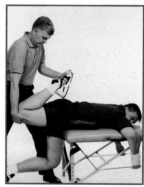
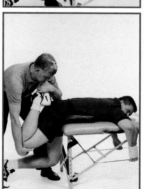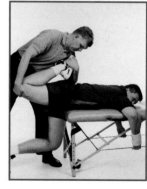

Method Part 1: From a prone position, patient should lean over a table, placing the resting leg as far forward along the side of the table as possible, weight free, with the upper body and pelvis resting firmly on the surface. Ask subject to flex the knee, moving the lower leg toward the buttocks to help release the proximal rectus femoris which assists in hip flexion. The proximal end is often the tightest portion of the muscle. Release the foot to the 90 degree starting position and repeat.

Repetitions: One or two sets of 10.

Method Part 2: Ask the subject to flex his/her exercising leg as far as possible and adduct it toward the opposite thigh. Clasp the ankle with your near side hand, placing your elbow across pelvis. A seat belt may be used to help stabilize pelvis. Then ask subject to initiate movement by contracting the gluteus maximus and hamstrings to move thigh backwards. Help the stretch with controlled guidance and gentle aid at end of movement. Release and repeat. Alternate legs after each set.

Repetitions: Two sets of 10.

HIP EXTERNAL ROTATOR STRETCH: PRONE

Muscles Stretched: External rotators, including, obturator externus, inferior gemellus, obturator internus, superior gemellus, piriformis muscle.

Muscles Contracted: Internal rotators — gluteus minimus, gluteus medius, pectineus, tensor fascia latae.

Introduction: This stretch is intended for isolation of each individual external hip rotator muscle. When external rotators of the hip are tight, the restricted muscles limit lateral quickness and ability to change direction.

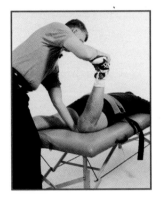 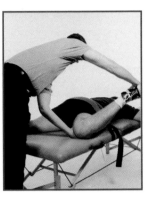

Method: The pelvis must be stabilized with one or two seat belts to prevent pelvis movement. Ask subject to assume a prone position with knee flexed at 90 degrees. As subject contracts the internal rotators, move his/her lower thigh away from midline and move lower leg laterally away from midline to stretch the deep external rotators. Therapist will assist at end of movement. Moving the thigh medially (inward) will stretch the distal positioned quadratus femoris muscle. Return to starting position.

Repetitions: 8-10.

Specific Stretches: From this basic position, other muscles can be stretched for each additional 10 degrees the thigh is moved away from midline Abducting the thigh an additional 10 degrees away from midline isolates each specific lateral rotator muscle in the order following: obturator externus muscle, inferior gemellus muscle, obturator internus muscle, superior gemellus muscle, piriformis muscle. To achieve these additional stretches, the therapist-trainer should place his/her outer hand along inside of ankle while inner hand assists the subject during internal rotation of the femur to help prevent strain of the medial collateral ligament of the knee.

Caution: Use precaution so knee is not strained or hip overstretched by too much pressure. Return to starting position.

Repetitions: One or two sets of 10 for each angle.

HIP EXTERNAL ROTATOR STRETCH: SUPINE

Muscles Stretched: Six deep external rotators — quadratus femoris, obturator externus, inferior gemellus and piriformis muscles, and outer gluteus maximus.

Muscles Contracted: Gluteus medius, gluteus minimus, and tensor fascia latae.

Introduction: This exercise is beneficial for movement flexibility and restoration of range of motion.

Method: Instruct the patient to place rope around midfoot and clasp with same side hand. Therapist should place opposite side hand above knee to stabilize femur. Instruct patient to rotate hip by moving lower leg away from midline. Assist at end of movement or have patient use rope and continued muscle effort.

Continued On Following Page

HIP EXTERNAL ROTATOR STRETCH: SUPINE (CON'T.)

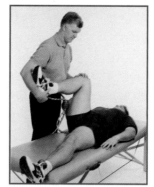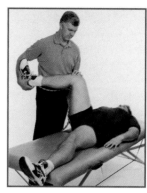

Compensation Check: Prevent compensation of pelvis, which will attempt to lift in direction of lower leg movement, by spreading leg (abduct) wide and turning outward. Therapist may stabilize pelvis using a seatbelt.

Additional Stretches: When thigh is closest to midline, the quadratus femoris receives greatest isolation. From this basic position, the following list of muscles can be stretched for every additional 10 degrees of thigh abduction: obturator externus, inferior gemellus, obturator internus, superior gemellus, and piriformis.

Repetitions: One or two sets of 10 for each angle.

HIP EXTERNAL ROTATOR STRETCH: SITTING

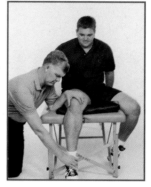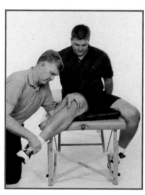

Muscles Stretched: Gluteus maximus and six deep external rotators.

Muscles Contracted: Gluteus minimus, pectinius and tensor fascia latae.

Introduction: Stretching these muscles results in increased lateral movement and quickness.

Method: Ask subject to sit at the edge of the table and place a pad or firmly rolled towel under the knees. Instruct him/her to keep buttocks on table throughout movement. Subject should move lower leg away from midline with assistance at end of movement. Release and repeat. Alternate legs after each set.

Additional Stretch: Move thigh away (abduct) from midline an additional 10 degrees for each external rotator muscle to be isolated. (See previous stretch.)

Compensation Check: Do not allow same side of pelvis to hike upward.

Repetitions: Two sets of 10.

HIP INTERNAL ROTATOR STRETCH: PRONE

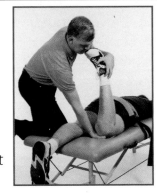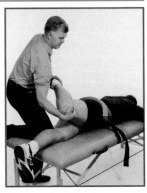

Muscles Stretched: Tensor facia latae, gluteus medius, gluteus minimus, and psoas major.

Muscles Contracted: Six external rotators-obturator internus, obturator externus, gemellus superior, gemellus inferior, quadratus femoris, piriformis, and gluteus maximus.

Method: Subject assumes a prone position with the therapist standing to the side facing him/her. Stabilize the pelvis with a seat belt and position subject's noninvolved leg across midline. The muscles being lengthened will depend on the angle of approach. Place one hand near inside of lower thigh-knee. The opposite hand is placed on outside of lower leg. From the initial position rotate the hip outward to stretch the gluteus medius and tensor fascia latae.

Specific Stretches: Extend the hip 5 degrees and hyperadduct 5 degrees to isolate the gluteus minimus. Isolate the psoas by hyperextending and adducting an additional 5 degrees. For isolation of the sacral-coccyx muscles and sacro tuberous ligament, hyperextend and hyperadduct the hip as far as possible and then externally rotate.

Notes: The number of repetitions at each angle will depend on the tissue limitations at each angle.

Repetitions: One or two sets of 10.

HIP INTERNAL ROTATION STRETCH : SUPINE

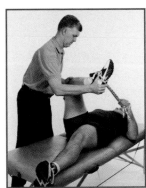

Muscles Stretched: Gluteus medius gluteus minimus, and tensor fascia latae.

Muscles Contracted: Obturator internus, obturator externus, gemellus superior, gemellus inferior, quadratus femoris, and piriformis and gluteus maximus.

Method: From a supine position, the patient should flex his/her hip and knee joints to a 90 degree angle. Stabilize the pelvic girdle with a seat belt. Initially the knee is positioned vertically. Places one hand near the inside of the lower thigh-knee and the opposite hand on the outside of lower leg. From this position, ask subject to contract the six deep external rotators by moving the exercising leg across midline. Use your hand to assist or instruct patient in use of rope for assistance.

Specific Stretches: Adduct the femur across the midline an additional 10 degrees to isolate the gluteus minimus, continue 10 degrees farther to stretch the psoas. Adducting maximally and externally rotating the hip will isolate the sacral-coccyx muscles and sacro-tuberous ligament area.

Notes: Total repetitions will depend on the tissue elasticity at each angle.

Repetitions: One or two sets of 10 repetitions.

HIP INTERNAL ROTATOR STRETCH: SEATED

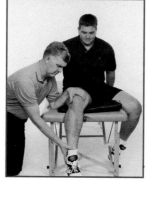
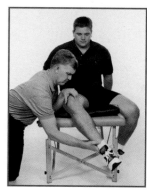

Muscles Stretched: Gluteus medius, gluteus minimus, pectinius, and tensor fascia latae.

Muscles Contracted: Gluteus maximus and six deep external rotators.

Introduction: Medial rotation may be limited following an injury or from inactivity.

Method: Place a pad or firmly rolled towel under the patient's knees and instruct him/her to keep buttocks resting on table. Ask subject to move one leg across midline. Assist at end of active movement. Release to starting position and repeat.

Additional Stretches: To isolate each muscle, move thigh 10 degrees farther toward midline. Each additional 10 degrees of movement toward midline will enable greater individual internal hip rotator isolation. Alternate legs at end of each set.

Compensation Check: Do not allow opposite side of pelvis to hike upward.

Repetitions: One or two sets of 10.

GLUTEUS MAXIMUS STRETCH

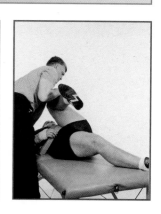

Muscles Stretched: Lower back rotators, outer hip, and especially gluteus maximus muscle.

Muscles Contracted: Hip flexors, abdominals, medial hip rotators, and hip adductors.

Introduction: This is a gentle stretch for lower back and hip flexibility problems.

Method: From a supine position, subject should stabilize pelvis by moving nonexercising leg across midline and rotating same leg to inward extreme. A pad and seat belt also may be used to help stabilize pelvis. Ask patient to contract hip flexors, abdominals, medial hip rotators, and hip adductors by moving exercising leg towards bottom of opposite side breast. Subject may learn to assist stretch with both hands on outside of knee. Assistant should help subject with stretch and maintain position of noninvolved leg. Return to starting position following each repetition.

Repetitions: One or two sets of 10.

FIGURE 4 ROTATOR (PIRIFORMIS) STRETCH

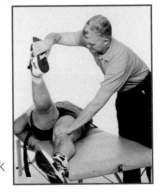
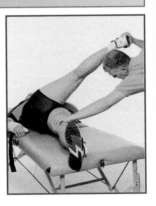

Muscles Stretched: Maximum stretch of low back rotators, gluteus maximus, gluteus medius and external hip rotator muscles. This is an especially good stretch for the piriformis muscle.

Muscles Contracted: Lower abdominals, internal hip rotators, and hip adductors.

Introduction: This is an important stretch for those with back histories, for releasing pelvic distortions and pressure on the hip, and for helping to free sciatic plexus nerve pressure (sciatica). It is also important for those who wish to improve quickness and lateral movement.

Method: From supine position, subject should rotate nonexercising leg inward and hyperadduct across midline as far as possible to help stabilize pelvis and isolate muscles to be stretched. A seatbelt may be used to help keep pelvis stabilized. Instruct subject to stretch opposite side by extending knee to within 10 degrees of full extension, lifting leg upward to as near a vertical position as possible (80 to 90 degrees). Ask subject to reach across his/her body as far as possible with scapulae (shoulder blades) and pelvis remaining on surface. Therapist should place one hand above knee on nonexercising leg to maintain maximal internal hip rotation and pelvic stabilization, and the opposite hand should assist the exercising leg to maximal stretch. Release, return to starting position, and repeat.

Repetitions: One or two sets of 10 depending on individual needs.

MEDIAL HIP-THIGH MUSCLE STRETCH

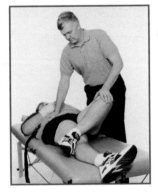
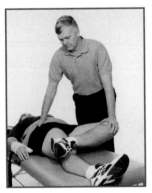

Muscles Stretched: Gluteus minimus, gluteus medius, pectinius, psoas, iliacus, gracilis, adductor magnus, adductor longus, and adductor brevis.

Muscles Contracted: Six deep external rotators and gluteus maximus.

Introduction: This stretch is important in the evaluation of people with lower back involvement, and it is very beneficial in freeing pressure on the lumbar spine.

Method: From the supine position, have patient flex one knee 90 degrees. Place lower leg on top of resting thigh just above knee. Place a thick foam pad or large folded towel on top of lower thigh to lessen pressure on extended leg. Normally the lateral region of the flexed leg should be able to touch the surface without moving the far side of the pelvis off the table. Stabilize the pelvis with a seatbelt and a pad or hold down the opposite side of the pelvis with your hand. Instruct the patient to attempt moving the thigh toward the surface. Carefully assist at the end of movement, release to starting position, and repeat.

Additional Stretches: Moving thigh closer to opposite resting thigh an additional 5 degrees a few degrees will isolate a different muscle.

Notes: Instruct the patient to contract the abdominals, to prevent lumbar spine hyperextension.

Repetitions: Two sets of 10 each side.

TRUNK FLEXIBILITY: ASSISTED

Maintenance of trunk flexibility is important in sports for injury prevention and for the development of maximum power and quickness. The restoration of trunk flexibility is also important following an injury or surgery. Movement limitations of the thoracic (mid back) and lumbar (lower back) including flexion, extension, lateral flexion, and rotation may limit spinal posture and lead to muscle pulls or more serious spinal injuries. Shortened muscles of the trunk and hip limit free pelvic movement.

SINGLE LEG PELVIC TILT

Muscles Stretched: This Williams Back Exercise helps attain maximum flexibility of the sacrospinalis (low back), proximal hamstring tissue, and gluteus maximus.

Muscles Contracted: Hip flexor and abdominal muscles.

Caution: If condition is postoperative, there is disc involvement, or there is severe pain, ask patient to flex the nonexercising knee 25 or more degrees. Otherwise, the nonexercising knee may remain straight and in contact with the surface.

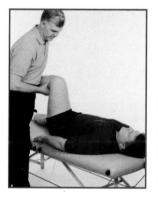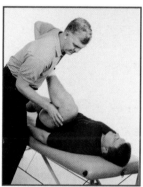

Method: From a supine position, ask subject to flex the exercising knee and pull it toward the axilla (arm pit) by contraction of the hip flexor and abdominal muscles. Subject may place hands behind the thigh to prevent pressure on the knee and provide slight assistance at the end of free movement. Therapist should assist by placing distal hand under the foot of subject's active leg and the proximal hand under the mid to lower thigh. Ask subject to move knee toward the axilla (arm pit) because moving the thigh toward the chest is limited by the stomach, chest, and hip joint at that angle. Release to starting position and repeat.

Repetitions: One or two 10 each side.

DOUBLE LEG PELVIC TILT

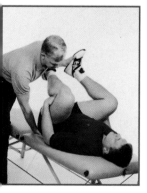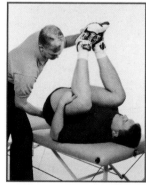

Muscles Stretched: Gluteus maximus and sacrospinalis (low back) muscles.

Muscles Contracted: Hip flexors and abdominal muscles.

Method: Subject should begin with knees and hips flexed at a 90 degree angle and thighs pointed vertical. Instruct subject to exhale and contract hip flexors and abdominal muscles, pulling the thighs toward the axilla (arm pits). Subject may place hands under the thighs and assist the contracting muscles in the stretching movement. Assist subject's active effort by placing the proximal hand under the pelvis and the distal hand under the feet with each repetition. Return to the starting position (thighs vertical) and attempt to move closer to the axilla.

Repetitions: 10.

BENT KNEE TRUNK FLEXION

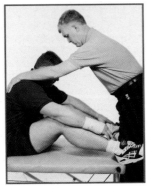 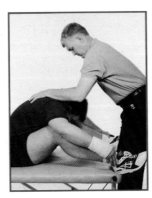

Muscles Stretched: Erector spinae and sacrospinalis muscles.

Introduction: Use care if subject's back has been injured or surgically repaired or if he/she is inflexible.

Method: Subject should be seated with knees flexed 4 to 6 inches. Instruct him/her to tuck chin, exhale, and firmly contract the abdominals as he/she curls body forward. You may place hand gently on upper mid-back and assist for 1 to 2 seconds. Release to the starting position and repeat. Do not let subject bounce, make rapid movements at the end of the active stretch, or hold the stretch too long.

Caution: It is dangerous to use your entire body weight to assist.

Repetitions: 10-15.

LUMBAR-SACRAL SPINE STRETCH

Muscles Stretched: Distal erector spinae and sacral-coccyx muscles.

Muscles Contracted: Cervical flexors, upper rectus abdominus, and internal and external oblique muscles.

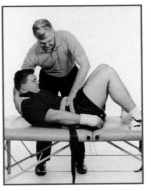 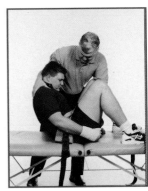

Introduction: The lumbar spine can be stretched safely and effectively when the pelvic girdle is stabilized by tilting the top of the pelvis backward. This movement is maximized by firmly strapping a pad across the top-anterior portion of the pelvis.

Method: Instruct subject to bend knees 4 to 6 inches and contract the lower abdominals to help stabilize the pelvis and then to tuck the chin, exhale and flex the cervical, thoracic, and lumbar spine. The therapist or assistant may help stretch the back muscles with gentle pressure of the hand on the back. The patient may provide active assistance with his/her hands by clasping the table or placing hands under the posterior thigh. Release to the starting position and repeat.

Notes: This stretch may be used in a very gentle manner for postoperative backs, backs with disc involvement, and other lower back disorders.

Repetitions: Two sets of 10.

LUMBAR- SACRAL SPINE STRETCH

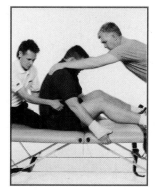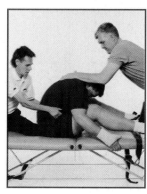

Muscles Stretched: Sacrospinalis distal attachments, erector spinae.

Muscles Contracted: Abdominals, internal obliques, external obliques, and hip flexors.

Introduction: This stretch usually follows Bent Knee Trunk Flexion and is an alternative to the Lumbar-Sacral Spine Stretch, one which utilizes a seat belt and pad.

Method: So that the lumbar spine and sacral-coccyx can be stretched safely and effectively, ask the subject to help stabilize the pelvic girdle by tilting his/her pelvis backward. Further stabilize patient by sitting behind the him/her to prevent the pelvis tilt. Instruct subject to flex knees 4 to 6 inches and contract abdominals, obliques, and hip flexors. Therapist should assist with hands at end of movement. Stretch, release, and repeat.

Repetitions: 10-15.

ADVANCED TRUNK ROTATION

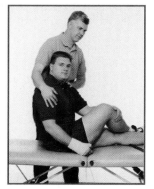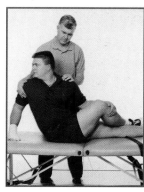

Muscles Stretched: Cervical, thoracic, and lumbar rotators.

Method: Ask subject to sit with one leg straight and to flex the opposite knee 90 degrees. Cross foot over and rest calf on the far side of straight knee or alternately to bend knees slightly and spread legs wider than hips. Subject should place opposite side elbow on outside of flexed knee and rest other hand behind his/her back. Instruct subject to turn head and trunk as far away as possible from midline. Therapist will stand at side of subject with hands placed on shoulders. At end of each movement provide gentle assistance. Release, face forward, repeat. Perform exercise on opposite side.

Repetitions: One or two sets of 10 each side.

THORACIC-LUMBAR ROTATION

Muscles Stretched: Rotators, erector spinae and sacrospinalis — muscles and connective tissue that may limit rotation of the thoracic-lumbar spine.

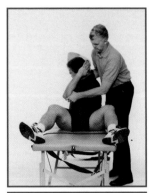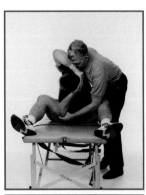

Muscles Contracted: Hip flexors, rectus abdominus external and internal oblique muscles.

Introduction: This stretch is especially important for people with scoliosis or back stiffness and for athletes of all sports.

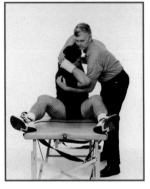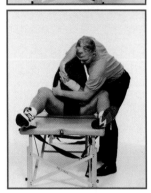

Method: Have patient take a seated position with his/her feet slightly apart. Hands are clasped behind head and knees are flexed 4 to 6 inches. Instruct patient to flex lower elbow close to opposite side of chest, tuck chin, exhale, contract abdominals, obliques and hip flexors and flex trunk forward (shoulder toward surface) as far as possible without bouncing. Help keep trunk rotated and assist gently at end of movement. Release, return to starting position, and repeat to same side. Instruct patient to exhale and flex trunk forward, bringing lead shoulder down between the knees toward the surface. Return to starting position, complete repetitions and change sides.

Notes: Some people may require an additional set of 10, as most people are tighter on one side.

Repetitions: 10 each side.

Muscles Stretched: Lateral spine flexors, quadratus lumborum (lateral), obliques, and erector spinae muscles.

Muscles Contracted: Same muscles opposite side.

Method: Therapist should instruct and assist subject to stand with feet shoulder width apart, knees fully extended, and pelvis horizontally level. Subject slowly leans lateral, directly over side of pelvis as far as possible. Therapist should help prevent lateral tilt of pelvis. Following completion of repetitions, subject should lean to opposite side extreme. Return to starting position and repeat.

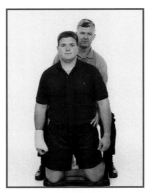
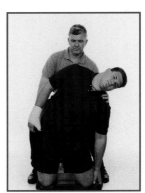
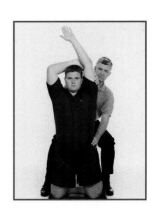
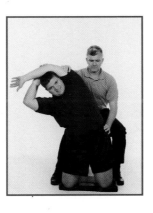
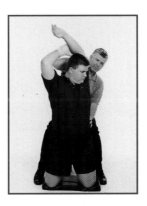
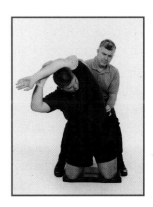

Additional Stretch: For greater isolation of the quadratus lumborum, rotate the trunk 45 degrees anterior without allowing pelvis to rotate. Move at a 45 degree angle obliquely in the direction front shoulder is pointed.

Notes: By placing the same side arm in a sideward elevated position (vertical), the serratus posterior and latissimus dorsi muscles receive greater stretch.

Repetitions: One or two sets of 10 repetitions for each side.

Muscles Stretched: Anterior portion of the thoracic spine and proximal abdominals.

Muscles Contracted: Erector spinae muscles.

Introduction: This stretch is especially helpful for the dorsal (anterior) thoracic spine and for those suffering from thoracic kyphosis (forward curvature).

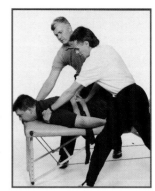 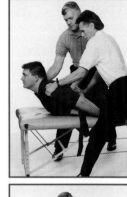

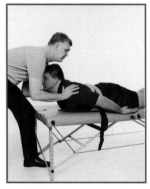 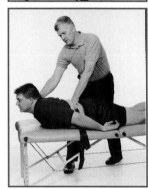

Method: Subject assumes a prone position, and therapist stabilizes the lower region of the thoracic spine by placing a pad and strap across the T9 to T10 region or by applying firm pressure to that area with the hand in a forward and downward direction. (It is necessary to prevent as much lumbar extension compensation as possible.) You may also place straps across ankles for greater stabilization. Once stabilized, ask subject to roll shoulders back and raise trunk as far as possible. Assist with your hands under shoulders or ideally, by having another assistant place hands under subject's shoulders while you prevent lumbar substitution.

Advanced Positions: As subject improves, you may increase strength to thoracic region by placing a sandbag across shoulders during the active effort.

Caution: Execute extreme care for those who may be suffering from osteoporosis or herniated disc.

Repetitions: Two or three series of 10 repetitions.

ANKLE-FOOT FLEXIBILITY: ASSISTED

Full range of motion of the ankle, subtalar, and metatarsal-phalangeal joints helps prevent injuries such as joint and muscle strains, and it helps relieve the effects of foot postural problems and postsurgical and aging factors. Improved flexibility also helps reduce recovery time in rehabilitation and increases sports potential. Assistance for stretching the ankle-foot areas may be necessary for those who are paralyzed, have just had surgery, are recovering from injury, or who have other limitations that prevent active involvement in the stretching process.

SOLEUS STRETCH: PRONE

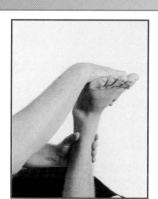
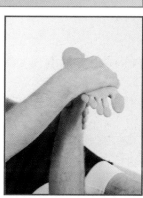

Muscles Stretched: Soleus.

Muscles Contracted: Anterior tibialis and extensor digitorums.

Introduction: Although a shortened soleus muscle or Achilles tendon is an infrequent problem, it sometimes occurs following injury or problems such as fracture, sprain, casting, or nerve damage.

Method: Patient assumes a prone position with the knee bent 90 degrees to prevent interference from the two-joint gastrocnemius muscle. If possible, have patient dorsal flex ankle with anterior tibialis and foot extensors. Assist patient at end of active movement, or if dorsal flexors are unable to move, therapist may passively stretch the soleus.

Caution: Be especially careful when working with patients with postsurgery Achilles tendon problems or who are paralyzed.

Repetitions: Two or three sets of 10.

SOLEUS STRETCH: SUPINE

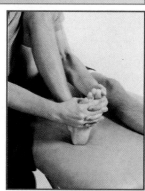

Muscles Stretched: Soleus.

Muscles Contracted: Anterior tibialis and extensor digitorums.

Method: Patient assumes a supine position, flexing knee 90 degrees, which prevents interference by gastrocnemius muscle. Have patient dorsal flex ankle with anterior tibialis and foot extensor muscles. Assist patient at end of dorsal flexion, or therapist may passively stretch the soleus if patient cannot dorsal flex ankle. For the passive stretch, brace your anterior shoulder or chest against subject's knee and interlock your fingers around ball of his/her foot. Assist at end of active movement or provide careful passive movement if he/she is paralyzed.

Caution: Be especially careful when working with patients with postsurgery Achilles tendon problems or who are paralyzed.

Repetitions: One or Two sets of 10.

ACHILLES STRETCH: PRONE

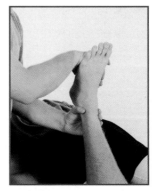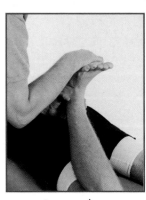

Muscles Stretched: Achilles tendon.

Muscles Contracted: Anterior tibialis and extensor digitorums.

Introduction: Because of injury, surgery, muscle disease, or temporary or permanent paralysis, the Achilles tendon may become shortened.

Method: Patient assumes a prone position with the knee flexed as far as possible to prevent muscle (soleus, plantaris, and gastrocnemius) involvement as the Achilles is stretched. Ask patient to dorsal flex ankle with anterior tibialis and foot extensors. Assist patient at end of movement or, if dorsal flexors are unable to move, passively stretch the Achilles.

Caution: Be especially careful when working with patients with postsurgery Achilles tendon problems or who are paralyzed.

Repetitions: Two or three sets of 10.

ACHILLES STRETCH: SUPINE

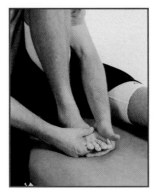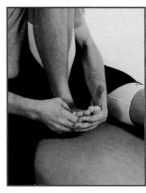

Muscles Stretched: Achilles tendon.

Muscles Contracted: Anterior tibialis and extensor digitorums.

Method: Subject assumes a supine position and bends knee as completely as capable, which permits greater isolation of the Achilles tendon. Have patient attempt ankle dorsal flexion (foot toward shin), by contracting tibialis anterior and foot extensor muscles, or if subject is unable to move actively, therapist can passively perform stretch. To accomplish this therapist should brace his/her anterior shoulder or chest against subject's knee and interlock fingers around ball of subject's foot. Assist at end of active movement or perform careful passive movement if the subject is paralyzed.

Caution: Exercise extreme care with postsurgery Achilles problems or if patient is paralyzed due to spinal cord injuries, stroke (C.V.A.), etc.

Repetitions: One or two sets of 10.

GASTROCNEMIUS (CALF) STRETCH

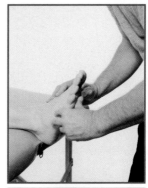
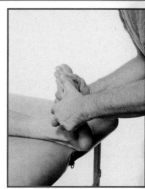

Muscles Stretched: Gastrocnemius.

Muscles Contracted: Anterior tibialis and extensor digitorums.

Introduction: This heel cord stretch lengthens the two-joint gastrocnemius muscle, reducing the risk of calf pulls, shin splints, Achilles tendon problems, and foot-ankle injuries.

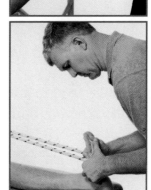
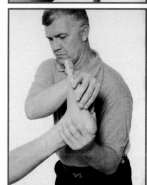

Method: Subject assumes a supine or seated position and fully extends the knee. Ask subject to dorsal flex the foot-ankle with anterior tibialis and foot extensors. Assist subject in pulling back the foot beyond the active range. As flexibility increases turn foot slightly inward to isolate outer gastrocnemius muscle and slightly outward to isolate inner gastrocnemius. Release and repeat. Encourage subject to do this stretch as often as possible alone or with assistance. Alternate legs after each set.

Repetitions: Two or three sets of 10.

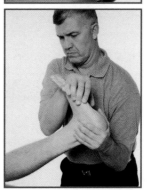
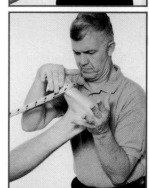

ANKLE INVERTOR STRETCH

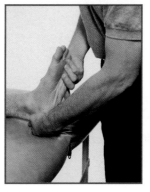
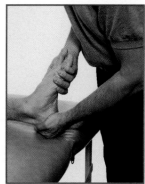

Muscles Stretched: Medial ankle muscles, including the tibialis posterior and anterior.

Muscles Contracted: Lateral subtalar and foot muscles, including the peroneus longus, peroneus brevis, and peroneus tertius and the extensor digitorum longus.

Notes: Patients with injuries, who have had surgery, or who have various muscle diseases or problems where movement is difficult or impossible, need assistance with this stretch. Subject may exercise from a seated, supine, or side-lying posture.

Method: With the patient's ankle at a near 90 degree angle as possible, attempt to turn subtalar joint (ankle-foot area) outward contracting the lateral subtalar and foot muscles. Subject should attempt to turn

Continued On Following Page

subtalar-foot outward as therapist gently assists motion with one hand around the heel and the other around the midfoot. Release and repeat from starting position.

Repetitions: One or two sets of 10.

ANKLE EVERTOR STRETCH

Muscles Stretched: Lateral tissue of the subtalar and foot regions including the peroneus longus, peroneus brevis, and peroneus tertius and the extensor digitorum longus.

Muscles Contracted: Subtalar and foot invertor (medial) muscles, including the tibialis posterior and tibialis anterior.

Notes: Patients with injuries, who have had surgery, or who have various muscle diseases or problems where movement is difficult or impossible need assistance with this stretch. Subject may exercise from a seated, supine, or side-lying posture.

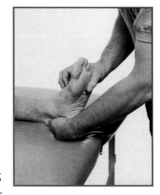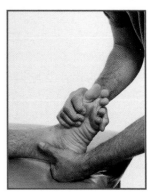

Method: Maintain patient's ankle at near 90-degree angle as possible, attempting to turn the subtalar (ankle-foot) inward. Subject should attempt to turn the foot inward as far as possible as therapist gently assists motion with one hand around the heel and the other around the midfoot. Release and repeat.

Repetitions: One or two sets of 10.

FOOT PRONATOR STRETCH

Muscles Stretched: Intrinsic dorsal muscles of the forefoot.

Muscles Contracted: Tibialis posterior.

Introduction: Prolonged periods of pronation or surgery and injuries to the toes and feet that require immobilization can cause the metatarsal-phalangeal regions to lose pliability, which in turn causes improper foot posture and results in foot stress or inadequate circulation.

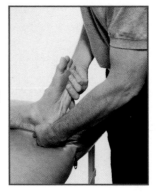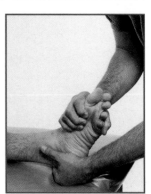

Method: Instruct subject in a mild plantar flexion position of the foot. Stabilize the heel with one hand to prevent movement and isolate the foot during supination. Have the patient attempt to move the foot inward as far as possible and assist stretch of the midfoot. Return to the neutral position and repeat.

Repetitions: One or two sets of 10, depending on condition of foot.

FOOT SUPINATOR STRETCH

Muscles Stretched: Intrinsic plantar muscles of the forefoot.

Muscles Contracted: Peroneus longus, peroneus brevis, and peroneus tertius and the extensor digitorum longus.

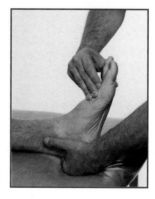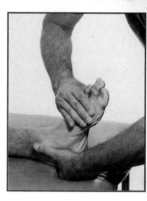

Introduction: Prolonged periods of supination or surgery and injuries to the toes and feet that require immobilization can cause the metatarsal-phalangeal regions to lose pliability, which in turn causes improper foot posture and results in foot stress or inadequate circulation.

Method: Instruct subject in a relaxed dorsal flexed position of the foot. Stabilize the heel with one hand to prevent movement and isolate the foot during pronation. Have the patient attempt to move the foot outward as far as possible and assist stretch of the midfoot. Return to the neutral position.

Repetitions: One or two sets of 10, depending on condition of foot.

DORSAL ANKLE STRETCH

Muscles Stretched: Tibialis anterior and extensor digitorum muscles.

Muscles Contracted: Plantaris, soleus, gastrocnemius, and flexor digitorum muscles.

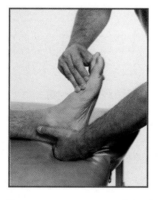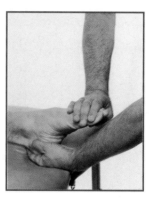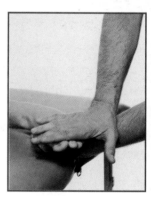

Introduction: Ankle plantar flexion (pointing the foot away from the body) may be limited because of injury, conditions causing weakness of the plantar flexors, or general lack of flexibility due to heredity, inactivity, or soreness. Over stress of these muscles may result in shin splints or tendonitis. Limited plantar flexion may be the result of a shortened tibialis anterior or tight fascia.

Method: Have subject plantar flex the ankle-foot downward (toes pointing toward the surface). Assist at end of movement.

Advanced Positions: Additional stretch of the anterior tibialis will be accomplished by supinating (turning inward and downward) the foot at the end of ankle plantar flexion. Release to starting position and repeat.

Repetitions: Two sets of 10.

METATARSAL ARCH STRETCH: EXTENSORS

Muscles Stretched: Metatarsal arch anterior, including extensor digitorum longus and brevis.

Muscles Contracted: Tibialis anterior to dorsi flex the ankle, flexor digitorum longus and flexor hallucis longus to flex all toes downward.

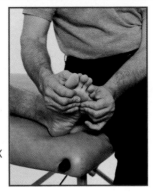 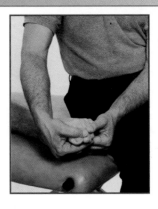 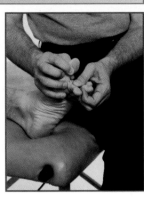

Introduction: This stretch is especially beneficial for people with limited flexion of the toes (hammered toes) and metatarsal arch region due to shortening of the dorsal (top) tissue.

Method: Have subject flex toes downward with active contraction of foot flexors. Provide gentle stretch with hands. Assist one toe at a time. Release and repeat.

Caution: These muscles and tendons will probably be quite sensitive, so proceed carefully.

Repetitions: Two or three sets of 10.

METATARSAL ARCH STRETCH: FLEXORS

Muscles Stretched: Flexor digitorum longus and brevis.

Muscles Contracted: Foot extensors including the extensor digitorum longus and extensor digitorum brevis.

Introduction: This exercise is beneficial for those subjects with

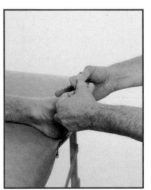 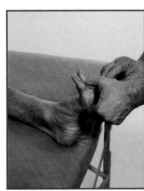

limited extension of the toes (hammered toes) and metatarsal arch region due to shortening of the plantar (bottom) muscles and connective tissue. Assistance may be required.

Method: Have subject attempt to extend toes upward with active contraction of foot extensors. Stretch one toe at a time, including great (big) toe. Stabilize on proximal side of distal joint with thumb and index finger to isolate distal phalanx. Following work with distal digit, stabilize proximal joint and assist proximal end of toe. With opposite thumb and index finger assist active movement.

Caution: These muscles and tendons will probably be quite sensitive, so proceed carefully.

Repetitions: Two or three sets of 10.

GREAT (BIG) TOE STRETCH (FLEXORS)

Muscles Stretched: Flexor hallucis brevis and flexor hallucis longus.

Muscles Contracted: Extensor hallucis brevis and extensor hallucis longus.

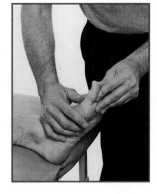 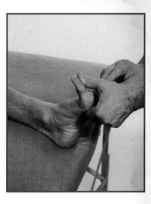

Introduction: This exercise is important when the arch is higher than normal, the big toe is hammered, or the foot has been affected by a neurological problem resulting in foot drop. In addition an inability to extend the great toe affects balance, coordination, speed, ability to push off properly, and length of stride. Athletes who do extensive training and wear foot orthotics that provide firm support, but limit foot movement, will lose foot mobility unless they consistently perform foot flexibility and strength exercises.

Method: Therapist should stabilize area just above proximal great toe joint with one thumb and index finger. Ask subject to extend big toe upward by contracting muscles on top of big toe. Therapist then gently assists with free thumb and index finger. Stretch and release. Beware of great tissue sensitivity.

Repetitions: Two sets of 10.

GREAT (BIG) TOE STRETCH (EXTENSORS)

Muscles Stretched: Extensor hallucis longus and extensor hallucis brevis.

Muscles Contracted: Flexor hallucis longus and flexor hallucis brevis.

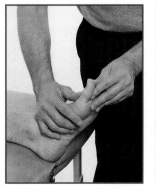 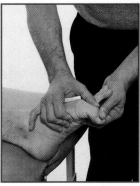

Introduction: Inflexible big toe extensors and tight Achilles tendon, soleus, or gastrocnemius muscles will lead to limited foot plantar flexion. A weak anterior tibialis muscle may also cause this problem. This will affect speed, balance, ability to push off properly, length of stride, and coordination. Conditions such as hammer toe, claw foot, metatarsalgia (chronic pain in the bones connecting the ankle to the toes), and abnormally high arch may result from limited great toe flexion.

Method: Ask subject to flex (bend) the big toe downward by contracting the muscles on the bottom (plantar surface) of the big toe. Gently assist the movement, remembering the muscle and tendon will be quite sensitive. Assist, release, and repeat.

Repetitions: One to three sets of 10.

GREAT (BIG) TOE STRETCH (ADDUCTORS)

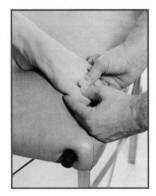 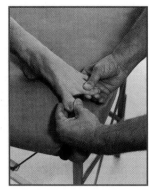 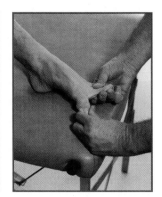

Muscles Stretched: Adductor hallucis, extensor hallucis longus, and extensor hallucis brevis.

Muscles Contracted: Abductor hallucis.

Introduction: Quite often we see a condition in which the largest toe is angled inward (hallux valgus). This condition may be uncomfortable and lead to formation of a bunion. The adductor hallucis muscle pulls the big toe towards the second toe. If the abductor hallucis is too weak to keep the toe in the normal neutral position, it will angle inward, especially if aided by the force of the shoe. Hallux valgus affects speed, balance, ability to push off properly, length of stride, and coordination. This stretch helps eliminate the inward angling of the big toe and helps prevent the major cause of a bunion. It also often positively affects a bunion that already exists by helping restore the posture of the big toe.

Method: Place slight pressure against the outside of the big toe and have the subject attempt to spread the big toe away from the other toes. Stabilize the four toes with your hand. Subject may be incapable of doing this movement actively without assistance. Assist subject's movement with thumb and index finger of free hand. (See previous Big Toe Extensor Stretch). **Additional Stretch:** Following stretching of extensors and adductors of big toe, do a combination stretch downward and outward with assistance, for maximum stretch of big toe extensors and adductors. Assist, release and repeat.

Caution: Be very gentle because sensitivity of the joint, muscles, connective tissue, scar tissue, or nerve ending will affect stretch. Do not be discouraged about results because joint and muscle distortion take time to correct.

Repetitions: Two or three sets of 10.

LITTLE TOE STRETCH

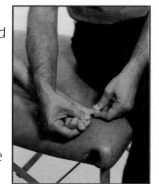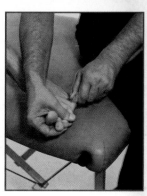

Muscles Stretched: Flexor digitorum longus, flexor digitorum brevis, abductor digiti minimi, plantar interossei, and flexor digiti minimi.

Muscles Contracted: Extensor digitorum longus, extensor digitorum brevis, and abductor digiti minimi.

Introduction: Frequently the little toe is postured in the shoe in a position of flexion, hyperadduction, and medial rotation. This fifth toe slides under the fourth toe rendering both functionally limited and placing greater stress on the medial foot and arches.

Method 1: The subject should attempt lifting the little toe upward, contracting the extensor digitorum longus. Isolate the affected area, placing the thumb and index finger proximal to the affected digit. Assist the active subjects effort with the remaining thumb and index finger.

Method 2: To stretch the adductor (web) portion on the toe, have the subject attempt to spread the toe while you stabilize the adjoining toe and assist in spreading of the little toe.

Method 3: If the toe is also rotating inward, mildly de-rotate toe in opposite direction.

Caution: Stretch slowly, as connective tissue will usually be very short.

Repetitions: Two or three sets of 10, according to the condition of the toe.

NOTES

CONTRAINDICATED OR QUESTIONABLE STRETCHING TECHNIQUES

When anatomical or physiological principles are violated, some stretching exercises may actually be irritating to the joints and muscles. There is potential danger from incorrect posture or from forces applied to vulnerable areas such as the neck, lower back, knees, or multiple joint muscles.

Tissues lengthen more readily when the agonist muscle group contracts and moves the joint in a shortening contraction (flexion) which enables the antagonist muscles and connective tissues to lengthen without active tension. If a muscle is performing a lengthening contraction, the lengthening muscles cannot simultaneously remain in a relaxed state. This endangers the safety principal of the myotatic (stretch) reflex. This action and the holding of the position for more than 1 1/2 to 2 seconds causes the muscles that are attempting to lengthen to receive greater tension as they hold the weight of the joint(s).

The myotatic (stretch) reflex functions as a safety mechanism. In a sustained, overpowering manner stretching in eccentric contraction violates the safety principles, representing a danger to the fibers being forcefully elongated.

The following exercises are contraindicated, in my opinion, for anyone seeking a safe, healthy stretching program.

HURDLE STRETCH: FORWARD FLEXION

From this position the hamstrings, gluteus maximus, back muscles, including the sacrospinalis and erector spinae, are in a lengthening (eccentric) contraction while you lean forward. In addition, the pelvis rotates, placing cross-plane force on the lower back. The long back muscles are forced to try to lengthen simultaneously with the hamstring muscles of the posterior thigh. See active bent knee trunk flexion and hamstring stretch, gluteus maximus stretch, bent knee and straight leg hamstring stretch exercises in the previous section of this book for safe and effective exercises that accomplish the same goal.

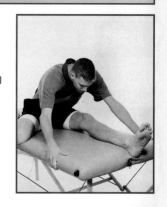

HURDLE STRETCH - HIP FLEXOR

The hip flexors, especially the rectus femoris (two joint muscle) and psoas major are placed in a stretch posture while doing eccentric contraction. The back is forced to hyperextend as the rectus femoris and iliopsoas contract. Too much stress is placed on the hip and lower back regions. This exercise may also irritate the anterior lower leg because the anterior muscles are also contracting. See active stretch exercise for psoas, rectus femoris, hip rotator, and ankle plantar flexion in the previous section to better stretch these areas.

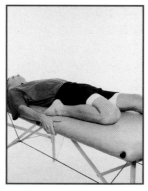
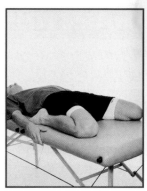

FRONT SPLITS

In the front split position the front leg muscles being stretched are the hamstrings (posterior thigh), hip adductors (inner thigh), and internal hip rotators all in eccentric contraction. The rear leg hip flexors (front thigh), external hip rotators, and lower back muscles are all in a state of eccentric contraction. See exercises for active hamstring, rectus femoris, psoas, hip adductor, and hip rotator for safe approaches to stretching the muscles involved in being able to perform a split.

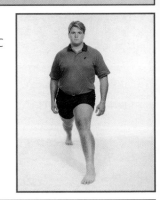

GROIN SINGLE LEG

The adductor magnus, adductor longus, adductor brevis, gracilis, and pectinius are in eccentric contraction as the subject lowers the body downward. Pressure is also placed on the medial hip rotators and psoas major, which causes pressure to the lower back.

See active hip adductor stretch (groin) in active section for safer approach.

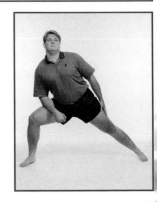

LATERAL SPLIT

This is a dangerous exercise that can cause groin (hip adductor) injury. Adductor magnus, adductor longus, adductor brevis, gracilis, and pectinius muscles on both sides are in eccentric contraction. The internal rotators of the hip and psoas major are also contracting with the lumbar spine hyperextending. This is potentially dangerous to hip and low back areas. See active hip adductor, psoas and hip rotator stretches in active section.

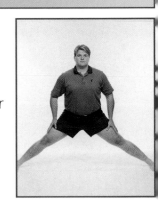

HAMSTRINGS

When you place your leg on a table, step or bar, the erector spinae, sacrospinalis, gluteus maximus, and hamstring muscles are in a state of eccentric (lengthening) contraction as the leg is lifted and held in position while the body leans forward. Pressure is placed on the back hip adductors, tensor fascia latae, and posterior thigh to elongate, which is made difficult by the working state of the muscles. See active exercises including bent knee trunk flexion, hip adductors, hip abductors and hamstring stretching in previous section.

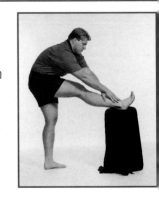

TOE TOUCHING

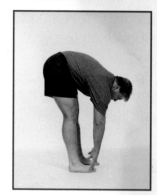

This stretch is especially bad for people suffering from lower back or hamstring problems. It is a composite movement involving all muscles of posterior body. The neck, long back, gluteus maximus, hamstring, and calf muscles perform a lengthening contraction to stabilize body segments. Pressure is placed on the back, hip, and lower leg areas. See active bent knee trunk flexion, hamstring, and gastrocnemius flexibility exercises to stretch safely.

Please note that this exercise may be used if the back, gluteals, hamstrings, and calves have been stretched previously and this is used as a secondary stretch later in a sports situation. In order to do this stretch successfully, contract anterior muscles of trunk, thigh, and lower leg and do not hold stretch position, instead repeat slowly 4 to 5 times.

BILLIG STRETCH

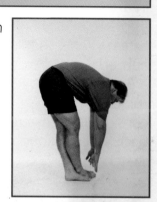

Touching the toes with the knees locked and legs crossed places a tremendous strain on the hamstrings, hip abductors, lateral hip rotators, gluteals, calves, lower back, and erector spinae back muscles. All these muscles are in the working status of a lengthening (eccentric) contraction. This exercise is especially contraindicated for people with back or hamstring problems. See active stretch exercises in the previous section including bent knee trunk flexion, thoracic-lumbar rotation, hamstring and gastrocnemius (calf) stretching.

CALF STRETCH

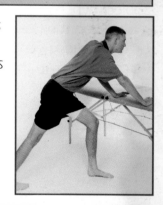

In a standing, forward lean posture the gastrocnemius, soleus, and plantaris muscles are involved in a lengthening (eccentric) contraction. The hamstrings and gluteus maximus muscles are also contracting to support the hip and knee joints. This means that while these muscles are contracting to support the knee and ankle joints from collapsing, we expect the same muscles to also be in a state of relaxation and passively stretch! This is more easily accomplished while seated as previously illustrated in the Active Ankle-Foot Flexibility section (i.e., gastrocnemius stretch and soleus stretches).

BANANA OR ROCKER STRETCH

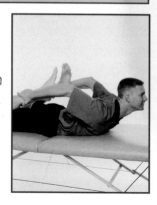

In the prone position the subject reaches back and clasps the ankle while simultaneously lifting the head and upper body. This is a dangerous exercise because the spinal muscles are contracting from both ends simultaneously. Posture that exhibit counter current (both ends contract toward the middle) movement may cause spasm or undue disk pressure. Unnecessary pressure is exerted on the back, hips and knees.

REVERSE TRUNK FLEXION

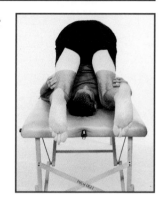

Beginning in the supine position the legs are lifted overhead until the feet touch the surface. In this posture the erector spinae and hamstring muscles perform lengthening (eccentric) contractions. There is unnecessary pressure placed on the cervical spine and thoracic spine, which may cause irritation or injury. Safe stretching exercises to stretch the hamstrings and long spinal muscles are located in the Active section of this book.

BACK STRETCH: SEATED

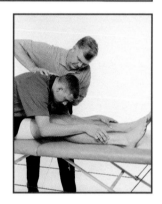

In a seated position, the subject sits with the legs extended and leans forward as far as possible. Occasionally an external force is applied by an assistant. Although external force should always be gentle and nonsustaining, this exercise is frequently applied with considerable prolonged force. The back and hamstring muscles, which are often inflexible, are in a state of eccentric (lengthening) contraction when the subject bends forward. This status and a prolonged external force, which is often considerable, may result in irritation or injury to the muscles or joints, specifically the back, hips, or knees. See the active or assistive sections for more effective and safer stretches involving bent knee trunk flexion and hamstring stretching.

NECK BRIDGE

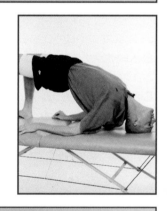

Subject hyperextends the spine and is in a posture where much of the body weight is borne on the head during movements of flexion, extension, lateral flexion, and circumduction. Considerable stress is placed on the cervical and thoracic spine. Forces placed on the cervical spine (neck) may lead to muscle strain or possible structural injury to the neck.

The cervical vertebrae and discs were not constructed to endure heavy weight bearing or shearing forces as evidenced by old sports and automobile injuries. See Neck Flexibility exercises in the previous section to develop increased strength and flexibility with greater safely.

HIP ADDUCTOR STRETCH

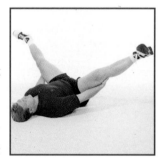

When stretching the adductors from the supine, the extended legs are stationed vertically above the hips. In this posture there is an attempt to stretch the adductor muscles (inner thigh) which include the gracilis, pectinius, adductor magnus, adductor longus, and adductor brevis. From the vertical position the subject spreads both legs sideward while the adductor muscles perform a lengthening (eccentric) contraction to support the pelvis and pelvis and femur. The psoas, rectus femoris, and medial hip rotators are contracting eccentrically. This is a dangerous exercise for the adductor muscles, which are frequently very tight. See adductor stretch in active section for proper technique.

GLOSSARY

Abduction: Movement away from the midline.

Active range of motion: Degrees of movement at a joint, movement caused by voluntary effort to move a body part being tested.

Adduction: Movement toward the body midline, opposite of abduction.

Agonists: Muscles whose active contraction causes movement of a part of the body. The contraction of the agonist muscle, also called the prime mover, is associated with the relaxation of its opposing antagonist muscle.

Antagonists: Muscles whose action (contraction) opposes that of the agonist muscles. Antagonist muscles relax to allow the agonists to effect movement.

Anterior: Front of the body or front of a body part.

Anterior pelvic tilt: Forward tilt of pelvis, which tends to increase lumbar curve (lordosis).

Circumduction: A movement that includes flexion, abduction, extension, and adduction performed in sequence.

Concentric (contraction): Movement during contraction as the muscles shorten.

Contracture: Sustained intrinsic activation that causes muscle shortening absent of motor unit action potentials.

Depression: Gliding motion in which the scapula moves downward. Opposite of elevation.

Dorsiflexion: To lift or flex the foot so that the toes are elevated.

Eccentric Contraction: Contraction during which the muscle lengthens.

Elevation: Gliding motion in which shoulder blade (scapula) moves upward. Opposite of shoulder girdle depression.

Extension: A motion in which two parts of the body on either side of a joint are moved farther away from each other.

Extensor: A muscle that extends or enlarges a joint angle.

Eversion: The motion of turning the foot outward on the talus and the front of the foot on the rear of the foot at the transverse tarsal joint.

Continued On Following Page

External rotation: A movement that is lateral or away from the body.

Flexion: The motion of bending or the state of being bent; also decreasing the angle.

Flexors: Any muscle that flexes or closes the angle of a joint in the human body.

Forefoot: The portion of the foot in front of the transverse tarsal (ankle) joint.

Hallux valgus: Condition in which the first (great) toe is positioned inward towards the other four toes.

Hammer toe: Chronic flexion of the interphalangeal joint of the big toe or of the proximal interphalangeal joints of the smaller toes.

Horizontal abduction-extension: A position in which the arms are shoulder high and the palms are together; the hands separate, moving apart horizontally in back of the chest.

Horizontal flexion: The motion of bringing the arm closer to the front of the chest from a starting position at 90 degrees of abduction from the shoulder.

Hyperextension: The extension of a limb or body part beyond its normal range of motion or backwards beyond 0 degrees. Especially prevalent in the neck, back, shoulder, hip, or wrist.

Internal rotation: Horizontal movement of a limb toward the body; medial or inward rotation.

Intrinsic muscle: A muscle that is contained entirely within the organ or part it acts upon.

Inversion: Supination or the inward movement of the entire foot.

Kyphosis: Increased flexion or forward bending of the thoracic spine.

Lateral: A location farther from the middle of the body or away from the side.

Lateral rotation: External rotation of an anterior surface of the body away from the midsagittal plane.

Lateral pelvic tilt: Position in which the pelvis is tilted toward the lower side. One anterior-superior spine is higher than the other.

Lordosis: An abnormal extension increase in the curvature of the lumbar or cervical spine.

Lumbar spine: Lower back; spinal area above pelvic girdle.

Medial: Toward the midline.

Medial rotation: The motion in which the anterior surface of a body part is turned toward the midsagittal plane of the body; inward rotation.

Continued On Following Page

Passive range of motion: Degrees of motion of an anatomical joint when movement is produced by an outside force without voluntary assistance.

Pelvic rotation: Movement of the pelvis in the transverse plane about the body's long axis.

Plantar flexion: Bending the toes or the foot downward.

Posterior pelvic tilt: The cephaled (top) portion of the pelvis is shifted backward, resulting in a decreased curvature of the lumbar spine.

Pronation: The turning of a body part from the anatomical position (face up) 180 degrees to the opposite position.

Rotation: Movement of a structure around its axis.

Sciatica: Inflammation or impingement of the sciatic nerve that contributes to pain in the low back, hip, and leg.

Scoliosis: Lateral deviation of the spinal column.

Spasm: Increased tonicity of a muscle as a result of a involuntary muscle action.

Supination: The inversion and adduction of a body part, for example, when the sole of the foot or palm of the hand faces upward.

Valgus: Condition in which a body part is bent outward or away from the midline of an extremity.

Varus: Deformity in which a portion of the body is bent inward or toward the body's midline.

BIBLIOGRAPHY

Alter, Michael. Science of Stretching, 1st ed. Champaign: Human Kinetics, 1988.

Anderson, Robert A. Stretching, 1st ed. Bolinas: Shelter, 1980.

Anheim, Daniel D. Dance Injuries: Their Prevention and Care, St. Louis: The C.V. Mosby Company, 1975.

Basmajian, John V. Therapeutic Exercise, 5th ed. Baltimore/London: Williams and Wilkins, 1990.

Beaulieu, John E. Stretching for All Sports, Pasadena: Athletic Press, 1980.

Calais-Germain, Blandine. Anatomy of Movement, Seattle: Eastland Press, 1993.

Floyd, R.T. and Thompson, Clem W. Manual of Structural Kinesiology, St. Louis: Mosby, 1994.

Hungerford, Myk. Beyond Sports Medicine, Cosa Mesa: Sports Massage Training Instutute, 1993.

Kendall, Florence Peterson, P.T. and Elizabeth Kendall McCreary. Muscle Testing and Function, 3rd ed.
        Baltimore/London: Williams and Wilkins, 1983.

Klafs, Carl E. and Daniel E. Arnheim. Modern Principles of Athletic Training, 8th ed.
        St. Louis: C.V. Mosby, 1992.

Mattes, Aaron L. Flexibility, Active and Assisted Stretching, Sarasota: Aaron L. Mattes, 1990.

Norkin, Cynthia C. and Pamela K. Levangie. Joint Structure & Function, 2nd ed.
        Philadelphia: F.A. Davis Company, 1992.

O'Donoghue, Don H. M.D. Treatment of Injuries to Athletes, 4th ed. Philadelphia: W.B. Saunders, 1984.

Rasch, Philip J. Kinesiology and Applied Anatomy, 7th ed. Philadelphia: Lea & Febiger, 1989.

Shelton, Robert E., Leonard O. Greninger and Aaron L. Mattes.
        Basic Exercise, Pre-Conditioning and Re-Habilitation, Iowa:
        Eddie Bowers Publishing Company, 1973.

Solveborn, Sven-A., M.D. The Book About Stretching, Tokyo:
        Japan Publications, Inc., 1989.

Sweigard, Lulu E. Human Movement Potential, New York:
        Dodd, Meade & Company, 1974.

Travell, Janet G., M.D. and David G. Simons, M.D. Myofascial Pain and Dysfunction,
        Vol. 1. Baltimore: Williams and Wilkins, 1983.

Travell, Janet G., M.D. and David G. Simons, M.D. Myofascial Pain and Dysfunction,
        Vol. 2. Baltimore: Williams and Wilkins, 1992.